Phonological disorders in children

Phonological disorders in children

Theory, research and practice

Edited by
Mehmet S. Yavas

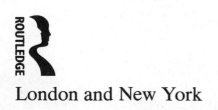

London and New York

First published 1991
by Routledge
11 New Fetter Lane, London EC4P 4EE

Simultaneously published in the USA and Canada
by Routledge
a division of Routledge, Chapman and Hall, Inc.
29 West 35th Street, New York, NY 10001

Typeset in 10/12pt Times Scantext by Leaper & Gard Ltd, Bristol
Printed in England by T.J. Press (Padstow) Ltd, Cornwall

British Library Cataloguing in Publication Data
Phonological disorders in children.
  1. Children. Speech disorders
  I. Yavas, Mehmet S.
  618.92855

  ISBN 0-415-05645-4

Library of Congress Cataloging in Publication Data
Phonological disorders in children : theory, research, and practice /
  edited by Mehmet S. Yavas.
     p.   cm.
  Includes bibliographical references.
  ISBN 0-415-05645-4
  1. Articulation disorders in children.   I. Yavas, Mehmet S.
  [DNLM: 1. Speech Disorders—in infancy & childhood.   2. Speech
Therapy—in infancy & childhood.   WM 475 P5737]
RJ496.S7P466   1991
618.92′855—dc20
DNLM/DLC
for Library of Congress   90-9028
                                              CIP

Contents

Notes on contributors

Pamela Grunwell is Head of the Department of Speech Pathology and Chair of Clinical Linguistics at Leicester Polytechnic, UK. She has published extensively on clinical phonology. Her publications include *The Nature of Phonological Disability in Children* (1981), *Clinical Phonology* (revised edition 1987) and *Phonological Analysis of Child Speech* (1985)

Barbara W. Hodson teaches at the Department of Communicative Disorders and Sciences at Wichita State University, in Kansas, USA. She has written extensively on phonological disorders. Her publications include *Targeting Intelligible Speech* (2nd edition, 1991) (with E. Paden), and *The Assessment of Phonological Processes* (revised edition 1986).

Eeva Leinonen is Senior Lecturer in Linguistics at Hatfield Polytechnic, UK.

Eva Magnusson teaches at Lund University in Sweden. She has written several articles on normal and disordered language, linguistic awareness and development of reading. Her publications include *The Phonology of Language Disordered Children: production, perception and awareness* (1983).

Susanna Evershed Martin teaches at the Department of Clinical Communication Studies at City University, London, UK.

Richard G. Schwartz teaches at Purdue University in Indiana, USA. He has written extensively on normal and disordered child language.

Carol Stoel-Gammon teaches at the department of Speech and Hearing Sciences at the University of Washington in Seattle, USA. She has published extensively on normal and disordered child phonology. Her most influential work (with C. Dunn) is *Normal and Disordered Child Phonology* (1985).

Mehmet S. Yavas teaches at the Florida International University in Miami, USA.

Preface

This book is aimed at a representation of the recent developments in the area of phonological disorders in children. It addresses a gap in the literature for students and practitioners of speech pathology and communication disorders who wish to develop their understanding of current issues in the applications of phonology to disordered child speech. By dealing with various aspects of a wide range of issues, this volume has the aim of neither simply offering therapists theoretical statements, nor presenting therapy in a theoretical vacuum.

As a teacher and researcher in the area of phonological development and disorders, I have always felt the need of books of this nature. In compiling this volume my aim was twofold: first, I wanted to bring together linguists and speech pathologists who share the same concerns; second, I have always searched for a collection that reflects the American and European views on the subject. This healthy combination achieved in this volume gave the opportunity to cover a variety of topics. These include the implications of phonological development to disorders from a clinical–linguistic perspective and concerns over the methods and procedures of therapy. It also includes the important debates on less commonly discussed topics like metalinguistic awareness and the interaction among language components in relation to disordered speech. Nevertheless, I am aware of the omission of a number of topics which might also have been included. Yet, their inclusion would have made this project a much bigger one than I had originally planned.

The reader will notice that there are several unresolved issues in phonological disorders requiring further investigation. Given this, it is only natural that he or she may, at times, disagree with some of the opinions expressed in this volume. It is hoped that this book will stimulate further discussion on those unresolved issues where our understanding is limited.

I would like to express my gratitude to authors who have contributed to this book; only with their participation was it possible for me to set the objectives of this volume. I am extremely grateful for their co-operation.

Mehmet S. Yavas
Miami, USA, 1990

Introduction

Mehmet S. Yavas

The study of language disability engages the interest of practitioners in many fields. These include professionals in the fields of speech pathology, audiology, linguistics, psychology, education and medicine, who will contribute to our understanding of language disorders. The past two decades have witnessed a marked increase in interest among linguists, and the application of linguistic principles to the study of speech and language pathologies has thus grown considerably. Consequently, a new field of enquiry called clinical linguistics has emerged. One subfield of clinical linguistics, clinical phonology, is concerned with the sound system of disordered language.

Clinical phonology is the application of phonological investigation to speech pathology and therapy: the principles and procedures of phonological analysis provide frameworks for the description of data and form the basis for assessment. Three aspects of clinical work – assessment, diagnosis and treatment – rely crucially on phonological analysis. In order to have reliable and relevant assessments we need adequate descriptions of patients' speech. These lead to the identification of the defining characteristics of different types of disorders and to informative diagnoses of disordered speech. On the basis of these adequate descriptions and diagnoses, appropriate treatment strategies can be defined.

The importance of the application of phonology to the clinical setting stems from the patterned nature of deviant speech. Phonological disorders are not random sound errors, but, rather, deviations that are systematically organized. That is, disordered phonology is not a system without order, but simply a system whose patterning is not identical to that of the norm. In the clinic, information on the patterned nature of the disordered speech is crucial for arriving at an accurate diagnosis, and this, in turn, serves as the basis for effective remediation.

Complete analyses of aberrant phonological systems will probably lead to the development of new, more sophisticated diagnostic and therapeutic methods and procedures. As Lorentz states (1976: 32):

a logical central goal of speech pathology ought to be a general characterization of the nature of deviant phonological systems: how they are structured, how they change, and what general or specific restrictions determine the form and range of application of phonological rules. The greater the number of explicit, well-documented accounts of such deviant phonologies available for analysis, the more likely the eventual attainment of this goal becomes.

Ingram's classic (1976) work is significantly responsible for the current interest in linguistically orientated studies on disordered child speech. From the beginning of the present decade (Hodson 1980; Shriberg and Kwiatkowski 1980; Grunwell 1981, 1982; Crystal 1982; Edwards and Shriberg 1983; Magnusson 1983; Nettelbladt 1983) to more recent work (Grunwell 1985; Stoel-Gammon and Dunn 1985; and Elbert and Gierut 1986) many additional researchers have helped to establish clinical phonology as a field of enquiry and have contributed substantially to our knowledge in this area. In the meantime, linguistically based studies of deficient child speech, which were restricted to a few journals fifteen to twenty years ago have exploded beyond the traditional journals such as *Journal of Speech and Hearing Disorders, Journal of Speech and Hearing Research, Journal of Communication Disorders* and *British Journal of Disorders of Communication*, to more recent publications, such as *Language, Speech and Hearing Services in Schools, Journal of Childhood Communication Disorders, Seminars in Speech and Language, Topics in Language Disorders, Child Language Teaching and Therapy, Applied Psycholinguistics* and *Clinical Linguistics and Phonetics*, to cite a few. Thus, it is clear that the relevance of the theoretical foundations upon which the study of phonology is based has gained recognition as being central to the theory and practice of speech therapy.

As the importance of phonological theory to speech therapy is being acknowledged, the contribution of clinical phonology to phonological theory is also gaining recognition. The older view that clinical data provide merely secondary evidence to theoretical issues is no longer considered valid by many phonologists. Instead, they consider clinical phonology, on a par with loan phonology, contrastive phonology and sociophonological variation, to be an important testing ground for theoretical positions in phonology. Thus, for many if not for all, clinical phonology is not only the application of phonology to the diagnosis and treatment of disorders, but also, and equally importantly, a significant field of study shedding light on phonological theory.

The field of phonology has developed significantly in the era following the publication of *The Sound Patterns of English* (Chomsky and Halle, 1968; hereafter *SPE*) during the last fifteen or twenty years. A number of phonological phenomena that could not be adequately dealt with in the classic model of generative phonology (Chomsky and Halle 1968) have found more satisfactory treatment in other approaches. Among these is the syllable. The need to introduce units larger than the segment into phonological representations has gained widespread recognition. Autosegmental phonology, which was first advanced to account for tonal phenomena (Goldsmith, 1979) provided insight into the study of syllable-dependent processes in Kahn (1976); whose work, in turn, was an important precursor to Clements and Keyser's (1983) CV phonology. Another significant advance has been the treatment of stress. Unlike in *SPE* phonology, where stress was treated in a fashion parallel to the treatment of segmental phenomena, metrical phonology has dealt with stress and other prosodic phenomena in a more structured way (Liberman and Prince, 1977; Hayes, 1981, 1984; Kiparsky, 1981; Prince, 1983; Selkirk, 1984). Other developments have influenced the treatment of phonology across levels. Lexical phonology, developed by Kiparsky (1982, 1985), Mohanan (1982) and Kaisse and Shaw (1985), makes crucial use of the distinction between word phonology and phonology above the word. All of these new advances have been made accessible through a number of recent texts, such as Nespor and Vogel (1986) on prosodic phonology, Anderson and Ewen (1987) on dependency phonology, Hogg and McCully (1987) on metrical phonology.

It is a truism, however, that there has been a considerable gap between the developments in phonology and its applications in clinical settings. What is available for clinicians has been restricted to studies in the structuralist, classical generative and natural phonology frameworks. Consequently, we have not yet seen any use of the newer phonological models (with certain notable exceptions, such as Gandour (1981), Spencer (1984)), in this area. This is not unexpected, however, for in order to be applied, a model and its theoretical basis first need to be firmly established. Its application to other fields always requires a certain amount of maturity.

The focus of this book is phonological disorders in children. While there are, on the one hand, children whose speech disorders are clearly linked to pathological conditions that are obvious and detectable (e.g., cleft palate), there are also children who provide evidence of abnormalities in phonological development without any detectable organic etiology. In the case of the former type of children, we can observe both phonological disorders and articulatory (phonetic) problems. In the case of children of the latter type, however, there has been a shift from labelling their problems as 'functional articulation disorders' towards viewing them as 'developmental phonological disorders' (Grunwell, 1980, 1981), that is, disorders of organization rather than articulation. The traditional view that the analysis of misarticulated speech should focus primarily on the motor or phonetic components of sound production has thus been modified, and, instead, primary attention is being given to the phonological component of production. (This is developed in detail in the first section of Grunwell's chapter (Chapter 2).) The aim of this book is to address a gap in the literature for clinicians who wish to develop their understanding of current issues in the application of phonology to disordered speech. The authors whose work appears here are among those at the forefront of advances in the field of clinical phonology. Their contributions present a variety of issues in this field and represent the often differing American and European views.

We owe a great deal to Jakobson's landmark study, *Child Language, Aphasia and Phonological Universals,* for stimulating the current interest in studies of phonological development. This work was particularly instrumental in inciting the investigation of the relationship between phonological theory and phonological acquisition. Over the past two decades there have been numerous works (Stampe, 1969, 1973; Smith, 1973; Ferguson, 1975; Ferguson and Farwell, 1975; Ingram, 1978, 1988; Donegan and Stampe, 1979; Menn, 1980; Elbert *et al.,* 1984) showing the importance of phonological acquisition to phonological theory.

Besides such studies, the last fifteen years have witnessed an unusual explosion of interest in the relationship between normal phonological acquisition and phonological disorders. The principle behind the movement in this direction is that deficient phonological acquisition can be identified and examined only if we understand the emergence, usage and progression of phonology in normally developing children (Compton, 1976; Ingram, 1976, 1981; Parker, 1976; Singh, 1976; Weiner, 1979; Hodson, 1980; Shriberg and Kwiatlowski 1980; Grunwell, 1981, 1982, 1985; Edwards and Shriberg, 1983; Hodson and Paden, 1983; Irwin and Wong, 1983; Locke,

1983; Menn, 1983; Stoel-Gammon and Dunn, 1985; Preisser *et al.*, 1988).

In Chapter 1, Stoel-Gammon gives an overview of current theories of phonological development and relates these to our understanding of phonological disorders in children. She discusses what is required of a theory and evaluates six approaches: the structuralist (Jakobson, 1941/68), behaviourist (Mowrer, 1952, 1960; Olmsted, 1966, 1971), natural phonology (Stampe, 1969, 1973; Donegan and Stampe, 1979), prosodic (Waterson, 1971, 1978), cognitive (Ferguson, 1978; Macken and Ferguson, 1983) and biological theories (Locke, 1980, 1983). She points out that the major short-coming of current theories is that they tend to emphasize either common patterns or individual differences. They also tend to posit simplistic equations of similarities with a biological basis and differences with a cognitive basis. The author stresses the need for a broader model that can more adequately explain the common patterns as well as individual differences. Such a model must incorporate at least three major components: an auditory–perceptual component, a cognitive–linguistic component and a neuromotor–articulatory component.

One of the most important contributions of clinical phonology is to the assessment of the patient's speech. The comprehensive phonological description and its comparison with normal patterns will guide the work that follows. Ideally, in order to discover the systematic patterns in the child's phonology, we need a healthy sample of his/her speech. The most obvious technique to use would be the analysis of children's spontaneous utterances. Basing the analysis on spontaneous speech samples is, however, time-consuming, since extensive recordings are needed to get examples of, for instance, segments in varied phonetic contexts. Even if the speech sample is large, accidental gaps might still occur in the data. There are also difficulties encountered with natural conversational speech, as many disordered children are not very forthcoming. One further, critical problem is the glossability of the patient's speech. In many instances, disordered children's spontaneous utterances are very difficult to understand and thus are unglossable. Given such inadequacies of spontaneous samples, many researchers find it necessary to utilize a set of preselected elicitation materials to obtain a glossable sample for the analysis. The prerequisites of such a sample are given by Grunwell (1987: 266).

Having achieved the goal of a representative sample, the clinician moves to the analysis of this sample. Grunwell's chapter (Chapter 2) reviews the requirements of clinically applicable assessment procedures. Among the different theoretical frameworks of phonological analysis that have been applied as the basis for clinical assessment procedures (including generative phonology, distinctive features and natural phonology), natural phonology has enjoyed a great deal of popularity. Grunwell's chapter evaluates five widely known assessment procedures that use this framework exclusively or as one of their methods. These are Weiner's (1977) Phonological-Process Analysis, Shriberg and Kwiatkowski's (1980) Natural-Process Analysis, Hodson's (1980) Assessment of Phonological Processes, Ingram's (1981) Procedures for the Phonological Analysis of Children's Language and Grunwell's (1985) Phonological Assessment of Child Speech. More specifically, her evaluation deals with the following clinical prerequisites according to whether the procedures achieve one of the following:

1   provide a description of the phonological patterns of the child;
2   identify the differences between the normal phonological patterns and the phonology of the child;
3   provide a framework in which to indicate the communicative implications of the child's patterns;
4   provide a profile in which to evaluate the developmental status of the child's patterns;
5   facilitate the delineation of treatment aims and the planning of remediation programs;
6   identify and evaluate changes in a child's patterns in reassessment.

It is commonplace in linguistics to view language in terms of different levels (phonology, syntax, semantics, etc.); our analyses have reflected this view for a long time. Although there might be sound methodological reasons for such an approach, this separation has recently been questioned. Specifically, evidence has been accumulating not only that there are problems in the delimitation of those separate levels, but also that the strict separation of levels obscures significant interaction between them. This interaction appears to be extremely important for a full understanding of normal development and language disorders. Schwartz (Chapter 3) discusses the interactions between phonology and other aspects of language in phonological development and disorders. In his extensive review of recent developments on this topic he first discusses the co-ordination of development and of disorders across the components of language. Although there is considerable literature bearing on this topic, the author feels that the co-occurrence of deficits across levels has not received as much attention as needed for us to understand the full range of possibilities. This is explored in great detail in his discussion of on-line processing interactions and the influence of these inter-actions on immediate behaviour, as well as on the course of develop-ment. Schwartz's discussion centres mainly on the relationships between syntax and phonology and between the lexicon and phonology, the former of which is probably the most productive area for investigation. Research suggests that increases in complexity in one domain have a cascading effect on other domains of language behaviour in normally developing as well as disordered children.

After discussing the critical importance of such findings for our understanding of disordered speech, the author proposes the modifi-cation of assessment and treatment procedures to accommodate the relationship between phonology and other levels of language.

Another topic that is discussed frequently in the literature is children's metalinguistic awareness. The growing interest on this topic is partially motivated by the observation that there is an intimate relationship between metalinguistic awareness and literacy. The relationship appears to be especially strong between phonological awareness and learning to read. Many researchers (Bradley and Bryant, 1983; Tunmer and Nesdale, 1985; Juel *et al.*, 1986; Pratt and Brady, 1988) have argued that phonological awareness is a neces-sary (though not sufficient) condition for learning to read. It has been suggested that children who do not spontaneously develop phono-logical awareness should undergo a training programme before they are formally introduced to reading.

Children's metalinguistic awareness has also been discussed in relation to two other developmental areas: cognitive development and language acquisition. Hakes (1980, 1982) has proposed that the development of metalinguistic awareness is primarily due to the cognitive developments, conjointly termed 'metacognition', that take place around middle childhood; during this period, the child becomes aware of his or her cognitive processes and their results, and can manipulate them on a conscious level. Thus, Hakes establishes a close link between the development of metalinguistic awareness of children and their cognitive capacities. At the same time, there are those who approach the matter within the context of language acquisition. Clark (1978), for example, has argued that the development of meta-linguistic awareness is a gradual process that goes hand in hand with language acquisition. According to this view, even two-year-olds show some elementary level of metalinguistic awareness, as evidenced by children's monitoring of their own speech.

Studies on children's metalinguistic awareness have dealt mostly with normally developing children; little is known about the meta-linguistic capacities of language-disordered children. However, knowledge concerning the latter would be highly relevant for both assessment procedures and intervention programmes. In addition, metalinguistic awareness may well have a bearing on the literacy experience of such children. Furthermore, as Kamhi *et al.* (1985) point out, many language-assessment procedures and remediation programmes require metalinguistic judgements. Thus, there is a clear need for research in this area. Moreover, such research would also shed light on some controversial theoretical issues. If, for example, children who show normal cognitive development yet have language problems perform at a lower level than normal children on meta-linguistic tasks, this could suggest that metalinguistic awareness is a linguistic capacity more than a cognition capacity.

The literature available on the metalinguistic awareness of phono-logically disordered children is carefully reviewed by Magnusson in her state-of-the-art chapter (Chapter 4). Since most studies have dealt with the phonological awareness of such children, she concen-trates mostly on the awareness of words, syllables and phonemes. The literature Magnusson considers often shows conflicting results, which she attributes to the varying task demands across studies.

On the whole, phonologically disordered children perform more poorly than normal children on metalinguistic tasks. However, there is considerable individual variation, and there are even children who are more linguistically aware than normal children. Magnusson discusses at length several possible explanations for these observ-ations and leaves the reader with a clear understanding that the relationship between language ability and language awareness is a highly complex issue.

The assessment of disordered child speech has the aim of identi-fying the inadequacies of the phonological system. Such systems are characterized by the loss of contrasts, and thus restrict the ability of the child to signal meaning differences. The inadequacy is said to be either 'communicative' or 'functional'. Identifying the contrasts that are absent in the child's system, then, has a crucial role in planning of therapy, given that such contrasts are a priority for any effective treat-ment.

Leinonen's contribution (Chapter 5) deals with communicative or functional (in)adequacy and implications for the assessment and management of phonological disorders in children. Starting with the question of 'what it is in the child's phonological system that hinders interpretation by the listener', Leinonen reviews the factors discussed in the literature. These include homophony, variability, auditory distance of the adult target sound and its realization by the child and frequency of the abnormality. They also include considerations from the point of view of the listener, such as his/her ability to interpret meaning. Leinonen recognizes that the complete account of inadequacy of a phonological system requires considerations of the domains of human communication and pragmatics. However, she does not attempt to develop such a broad view of disability because of the unavailability of appropriate analytical and integrative frameworks for analysing the child's disability. For the present, we have to be content with models that deal with smaller components. To assess the child's system within a narrower framework, however, does not mean that we should accept the current approaches available to phonological disability. They are too limited. What is needed, is to extend the existing models without attempting the broad and unattainable account of disability. Leinonen has devised a means of assessing, from lack of contrasts, potential homonymy in children's lexical systems. From this measure of homonymy Leinonen explains how an index of functional adequacy or loss (FLOSS, as she terms it) can be derived. This measure, together with a means of predicting potential homonymy in lexical systems enables one to assess the functional (in)adequacy of phonological systems.

After explaining how to measure FLOSS and predicting potential FLOSS, Leinonen deals with the implications for phonological assessment and for the planning of treatment goals. The author concludes that while the assessment of functional adequacy is, without doubt, a well-motivated enterprise, there still remain necessary refinements for its practical applicability in clinical contexts.

Once we have a reliable assessment of the child's speech, explicitly principled therapy can be planned. Clinicians and researchers have continuously been in search of more effective methods of treatment of disorders. Traditionally, the methods have focused on the development of motoric skills and phonological (linguistic) problems have been overlooked. During recent years, however, it has been recognized that many disordered children have little difficulty with motoric production, but at the same time are not capable of using the sounds of the language according to its system. One of the most important contributions of phonology to the clinical context is the introduction of an organizational model in which speech is not viewed simply as a result of articulatory movements but is guided by phonological organization. Consequently, current approaches to treatment aim to establish phonological concepts (e.g., contrasts between sounds) rather than to attempt to establish motoric skills. As succinctly put by Grunwell (1983):

> the fundamental premise of phonological therapy must surely be that the changes in speech production need to take place not so much in the mouth but in the mind of the child. The aim of treatment is to effect cognitive reorganization rather than articulatory training.

As pointed out clearly by Grunwell (1987) and Stoel-Gammon and Dunn (1985), however, it is very important to distinguish between the aims of phonetic and phonological treatment: the diagnosis of the nature of the disability should be clearly made so that each individual patient receives effective therapy. For example, symptoms due to a phonetic disability (e.g., acquired dyspraxia) would require different treatment procedures from phonologically based disorders (e.g., acquired dysphasia).

There are basically two types of phonologically based treatment procedures: these are (1) distinctive-feature approaches, and (2) phonological-process approaches. Distinctive-feature approaches (McReynolds and Bennett, 1972; McReynolds and Engmann, 1975; Costello and Onstine, 1976; Weiner and Bankson, 1978; Blache *et al.*, 1981; Ruder and Bunce, 1981; Singh *et al.*, 1981; Toombs *et al.*, 1981; Weiner, 1981) make the assumption that the features taught in one contrast will generalize to other sounds carrying the same features. Similarly, in the phonological process approach, the assumption is that the remediation of one or a few processes can affect the correction of a group or groups of phonemes at one time (Edwards and Bernhart, 1973; Ingram, 1976; Weiner, 1979; Edwards, 1983; Hodson and Paden, 1983).

No matter what the unit of therapy chosen, features or processes, the clinician will have to decide about the techniques of phonological treatment. It is probably here that new research would be most welcomed. Hodson (Chapter 6) elaborates on the cyclic method that she has developed for English- and Spanish-speaking children. She describes the phases of selecting target patterns and selecting production-practice words, the structure of remediation sessions and the nature of remediation activities. She emphasizes the importance of developing cross-linguistic research in this area.

In some cases of disability the dichotomy between phonetic and phonological approaches of remediation has been controversial.

Evershed-Martin's contribution (Chapter 7) stresses the importance of the interaction between articulation, phonology and perception in the treatment of disordered children. Given that a balanced inter-action between all levels of speech and language processing is neces-sary for normal speech development, the author argues that any remediation that treats any one level of functioning as independent is inadequate. She contends that, while the boundaries between percep-tion, phonology and articulation are by no means fully clarified, in every case of output failure, therapy should address all three. She presents a case study, in which she explains how one can achieve a multidimensional approach to remediation with input training.

By dealing with various aspects of a wide range of issues, this volume has the aim of neither leaving therapists with simple theore-tical statements nor presenting therapy in a theoretical vacuum. It is hoped that it will help lead students and practitioners of speech pathology and communicative disorders to a fuller understanding of phonological disorders in children.

REFERENCES

Anderson, J.M. and Ewen, C.J. (1987) *Principles of Dependency Phonology*, Cambridge: Cambridge University Press.

Blache, S., Parsons, C. and Humphreys, J. (1981) 'A minimal word-pair model for teaching the linguistic significance of distinctive feature properties', *Journal of Speech and Hearing Research* 46: 291–6.

Bradley, L. and Bryant, P.E. (1983) 'Categorizing sounds and learning to read a causal connection', *Natura* 301: 419–21.

Chomsky, N. and Halle, M. (1968) *The Sound Pattern of English*, New York: Harper & Row.

Clark, E. (1978) 'Awareness of language: some evidence from what children say and do', in A. Sinclair, R. Jarvella and W. Levelt (eds) *The Child's Conception of Language*, Berlin: Springer.

Clements, G.N. and Keyser, S.J. (1983) *CV Phonology: a Generative Theory of Syllable Structure*, Cambridge, MA: MIT Press.

Compton, A. (1976) 'Generative studies of children's phonological disorders: clinical ramifications', in D. Morehead and A. Morehead (eds) *Normal and Deficient Child Language*, Baltimore: University Park Press, 61–96.

Costello, J. and Onstine, J. (1976) 'The modification of multiple articulation errors based on distinctive feature theory', *Journal of Speech and Hearing Disorders* 41: 199–215.

Crystal, D. (1982) *Profiling Linguistic Disability*, London: Edward Arnold.

Donegan, P. and Stampe, D. (1979) 'The study of natural phonology', in D.A. Dinnsen (ed.) *Current Approaches to Phonological Theory*, Bloom-ington: Indiana University Press, 126–73.

Edwards, M.L. (1983) 'Selection criteria for developing therapy goals', *Journal of Childhood Communication Disorders* 7: 36–45.

Edwards, M.L. and Bernhardt, B. (1973) 'Phonological analyses of four children with language disorders', unpublished manuscript from the Institute of Childhood Aphasia, Stanford University.

Edwards, M.L. and Shriberg, L.D. (1983) *Phonology: Applications in Communicative Disorders*, San Diego: College-Hill Press.

Elbert, M. and Gierut, J. (1986) *Handbook of Clinical Phonology*, London: Taylor & Francis.

Elbert, M., Dinnsen, D. and Weismar, G. (eds) (1984) *Phonological Theory and the Misarticulating Child* (American Speech and Hearing Association Monographs 22), Rockville, MD: ASHA.

Ferguson, C.A. (1975) 'Sound patterns in language acquisition', in D. Dato (ed.) *Twenty-Sixth Annual Georgetown Round Table*, Washington, DC: Georgetown University Press, 1–16.

Ferguson, C.A. (1978) 'Learning to pronounce: the earliest stages of phonological development in the child', in F.D. Minifie and L.L. Lloyd (eds) *Communicative Competence Cognitive Abilities*, Baltimore: University Park Press, 237–97.

Ferguson, C.A. and Farwell, C.B. (1975) 'Words and sounds in early language acquisition', *Language* 51: 419–39.

Gandour, J. (1981) 'The nondeviant nature of deviant phonological systems', *Journal of Communicative Disorders* 14: 11–29.

Goldsmith, J. (1979) *Autosegmental Phonology*, New York: Garland.

Grunwell, P. (1980) 'Developmental language disorders of the phonological level', in F.M. Jones (ed.) *Language Disability in Children*, Lancaster: MTP Press, 129–58.

Grunwell, P. (1981) *The Nature of Phonological Disability*, New York: Academic Press.

Grunwell, P. (1982) *Clinical Phonology*, Rockville, MD: Aspen.

Grunwell, P. (1983) 'Phonological therapy: premises, principles and procedures', *Proceedings of XIX International Association of Logopaedics and Phoniatrics Congress, Edinburgh.*

Grunwell, P. (1985) *Phonological Analysis of Child Speech*, London: Nfer-Nelson.

Grunwell, P. (1987) *Clinical Phonology* (2nd edn), London: Croom Helm.

Hakes, D.J. (1980) *The Development of Metalinguistic Abilities in Children*, Berlin: Springer Verlag.

Hakes, D.J. (1982) 'The development of metalinguistic abilities: what develops?', in S. Kuczaj (ed.) *Language Development Volume II: Language Thought and Culture*, Hillsdale, N.J.: Lawrence Erlbaum Associates, 163–210.

Hayes, B. (1981) *A Metrical Theory of Stress Rules*, Bloomington: Indiana University Linguistics Club.

Hayes, B. (1984) 'The phonology of rhythm in English', *Linguistic Inquiry* 15: 33–74.

Hodson, B.W. (1980) *The Assessment of Phonological Processes*, Danville, IL: Interstate.

Hodson, B.W. and Paden, E. (1983) *Targeting Intelligible Speech*, San Diego: College-Hill Press.

Hogg, R. and McCully, C.B. (1987) *Metrical Phonology*, Cambridge: Cambridge University Press.

Ingram, D. (1976) *Phonological Disability in Children*, London: Edward Arnold.

Ingram, D. (1978) 'The production of word-initial fricatives and affricates in normal and linguistically deviant children', in A. Caramazza and E. Zurif (eds) *The Acquisition and Breakdown of Language*, Baltimore: Johns Hopkins Press, 63–85.

Ingram, D. (1981) *Procedures for the Phonological Analysis of Children's Language*, Baltimore: University Park Press.

Ingram, D. (1988) 'Jakobson revisited: some evidence from the acquisition of Polish', *Lingua* 75: 55–82.

Irwin, J. and Wong, S. (1983) *Phonological Development in Children: 18 to 72 months*, Carbondale: Southern Illinois University Press.

Jakobson, R. (1968) *Child Language, Aphasia and Phonological Universals*, The Hague: Mouton. (Original work published 1941.)

Juel, C., Griffith, P.L. and Gough, P.B. (1986) 'Acquisition of literacy: a longitudinal study of children in first and second grade', *Journal of Educational Psychology* 78 (4): 243–55.

Kahn, D. (1976) *Syllable-based Generalizations in English Phonology*, Bloomington: Indiana University Linguistics Club.

Kaisse, E.M. and Shaw, P.A. (1985) 'On the theory of lexical phonology', *Phonology Yearbook* 2: 1–30.

Kamhi, A.G. and Koening, L. (1985) 'Metalinguistic awareness in language disordered children', *Language Speech and Hearing Services in Schools* 16: 199–210.

Kiparsky, P. (1981) 'Remarks on the metrical structure of the syllable', in W.U. Dressler, O.E. Pfeiffer and J.R. Rennison (eds) *Phonologica 1980*, Innsbruck: Insbrucker Beiträge zur Sprachwissenschaft.

Kiparsky, P. (1982) 'From cyclic phonology to lexical phonology', in Van der Hulst and Smith (eds) *The Structure of Phonological Representations I*, Dordrecht: Foris Publications: 131–7.

Kiparsky, P. (1985) 'Some consequences of lexical phonology', *Phonology Yearbook* 2: 85–138.

Lass, R. (1984) *Phonology*, Cambridge: Cambridge University Press.

Liberman, M. and Prince, A.S. (1977) 'On stress and linguistic rhythm', *Linguistic Inquiry* 8: 249–336.

Locke, J. (1980) 'The inference of speech perception in the phonologically disordered child, I, II', *Journal of Speech and Hearing Disorders* 45: 431–68.

Locke, J. (1983) *Phonological Acquisition and Change*, New York: Academic Press.

Lorentz, J.P. (1976) 'An analysis of some deviant phonological rules of English', in D. Morehead and A. Morehead (eds) *Normal and Deficient Child Language*, Baltimore: University Park Press, 29–59.

Macken, M.H. and Ferguson, C.A. (1983) 'Cognitive aspects of phonological development: model, evidence and issues', in K.E. Nelson (ed.) *Children's Language*, vol. 4, Hillsdale, N.J.: Earlbaum, 256–82.

McReynolds, L. and Bennett, S. (1972) 'Distinctive feature generalization in articulation training', *Journal of Speech and Hearing Disorders* 37: 462–70.

McReynolds, L. and Engmann, D. (1975) *Distinctive Feature Analysis of*

Misarticulations, Baltimore: University Park Press.

Magnusson, E. (1983) *The Phonology of Language Disordered Children: Production, Perception and Awareness* (Travaux de l'institut de linguistique de Lund 17), Lund: CWK Gleerup.

Menn, L. (1980) 'Phonological theory and child phonology', in G. Yeni-Komshian, J.F. Kavanagh and C.A. Ferguson (eds) *Child Phonology,* vol. 1: *Production,* New York: Academic Press, 23–41.

Menn, L. (1983) 'Development of articulatory, phonetic and phonological capabilities', in B. Butterworth (ed.) *Language Production,* vol. 2, London: Academic Press, 3–50.

Mohanan, K.P. (1982) *Lexical Phonology,* Bloomington: Indiana University Linguistics Club.

Mowrer, O.H. (1952) 'Speech development in the young child: the autism theory of speech development and some clinical applications', *Journal of Speech and Hearing Disorders* 17: 263–8.

Mowrer, O.H. (1960) *Learning Theory and Symbolic Processes,* New York: Wiley.

Nespor, M. and Vogel, I. (1986) *Prosodic Phonology,* Dordrecht: Foris.

Nettelbladt, U. (1983) *Developmental Studies of Dysphonology in Children,* Lund: CWK Gleerup.

Olmsted, D. (1966) 'A theory of the child's learning of phonology', *Language* 42: 531–5.

Olmsted, D. (1971) *Out of the Mouth of Babes,* The Hague: Mouton.

Parker, F. (1976) 'Distinctive features in speech pathology; phonology or phonemics?', *Journal of Speech and Hearing Disorders* 41: 23–39.

Pratt, A.C. and Brady, S. (1988) 'Relation of phonological awareness to reading disability in children and adults', *Journal of Educational Psychology* 80 (3): 319–23.

Preisser, D.A., Hodson, B.W. and Paden, E. (1988) 'Developmental phonology: 18–29 months', *Journal of Speech and Hearing Disorders* 53: 125–30.

Prince, A.S. (1983) 'Relating to the grid', *Linguistic Inquiry* 14, 19–100.

Ruder, K. and Bunce, B. (1981) 'Articulation therapy using distinctive feature analysis to structure and training program: two case studies', *Journal of Speech and Hearing Disorders* 46: 59–65.

Selkirk, E.O. (1984) *Phonology and Syntax: the Relation between Sound and Structure,* Cambridge, MA: MIT Press.

Shriberg, L.D. and Kwiatkowski, J. (1980) *Natural Process Analysis: a Procedure for Phonological Analysis of Continuous Speech Samples,* New York: Wiley.

Singh, S. (1976) *Distinctive Features: Theory and Validation,* Baltimore: University Park Press.

Singh, S., Hayden, M.E. and Toombs, M.S. (1981) 'The role of distinctive features in articulation errors', *Journal of Speech and Hearing Disorders* 46: 174–83.

Smith, N.V. (1973) *The Acquisition of Phonology: a Case Study,* Cambridge: Cambridge University Press.

Spencer, A. (1984) 'A nonlinear analysis of phonological disability', *Journal of Communication Disorders* 17: 325–48.

Stampe, D. (1969) 'The acquisition of phonetic representation', CLS 5

(Proceedings of the 5th Annual Meeting of the Chicago Linguistic Society), 443–54.

Stampe, D. (1973) 'A dissertation on natural phonology', unpublished doctoral dissertation, University of Chicago.

Stoel-Gammon, C. and Dunn, C. (1985) *Normal and Disordered Phonology in Children*, Baltimore: University Park Press.

Toombs, M.S., Singh, S. and Hayden, M.E. (1981) 'Markedness of features in the articulatory substitutions of children', *Journal of Speech and Hearing Disorders* 46: 184–91.

Tunmer, W.E. and Nesdale, A.R. (1985) 'Phonemic segmentation skill and beginning reading', *Journal of Educational Psychology* 77: 417–27.

Waterson, N. (1978) 'Growth of complexity in phonological development', in N. Waterson and C. Snow (eds) *The Development of Communication*, New York: Wiley & Sons.

Waterson, N. (1971) 'Child phonology: a prosodic view', *Journal of Linguistics* 7: 179–211.

Weiner, F.F. (1979) *Phonological Process Analysis*, Baltimore: University Park Press.

Weiner, F.F. (1981) 'Treatment of phonological disability using the method of meaningful minimal contrast: two case studies', *Journal of Speech and Hearing Disorders* 46: 97–103.

Weiner, F.F. and Bankson, N. (1978) 'Teaching features', *Language, Speech and Hearing Services in Schools* 9: 29–34.

1 Theories of phonological development and their implications for phonological disorders

Carol Stoel-Gammon

It is a well-documented fact that children learn to produce most of the sounds and sound sequences of their mother tongue by the time they are five or six years old. Though this feat has been observed by parents and educators for centuries, prior to the 1960s there were relatively few attempts to explain the phenomenon. Only the linguist Roman Jakobson, who was the first to relate phonological acquisition to phonological theory (1941/68), and the psychologist H.O. Mowrer, who viewed phonological acquisition as a skill best described in terms of a behaviouristic stimulus–response model (1952), had published works which could be considered theories of phonological development. In the last two decades, however, as interest in the field of phonological acquisition has increased, the number of theories has grown dramatically and now includes, among others, Stampe's 'natural phonology' theory (1969, 1973), Waterson's 'prosodic' theory (1971, 1981), the 'cognitive' theory proposed by Menn (1976) and Macken and Ferguson (1983), and Locke's 'biological' theory (1983).

Though each of these theories has its own set of claims and assumptions (see discussion below), they all share a common goal of attempting to explain the process of *normal* phonological development. Yet, we know that some children fail to learn the sound patterns of their native language by five or six years of age, in spite of normal cognitive and motor abilities. To date, no theory has specifically addressed the issue of abnormal phonological development; however, some of the current theories can accommodate atypical acquisition better than others. The purpose of this chapter is twofold: first, to give a brief overview of current theories of phonological development; and second, to relate these theories to our current understanding of phonological disorders in children. The chapter will be divided into five sections, as follows: (1) requirements of a theory;

(2) current theories; (3) the nature of disordered phonology; (4) the relationship of current theories and phonological disorders; and (5) suggestions for future theories.

REQUIREMENTS OF A THEORY

Before discussing the current theories of phonological development, it is useful to consider what should be expected of an adequate theory. In my view, it should fulfil the following requirements:

1   Account for the body of factual information we have gathered about phonological acquisition. To meet this requirement, the theory must account for the *general patterns* as well as the *individual differences* observed in the order of acquisition of speech sounds, the use of phonological strategies and the occurrence of phonological processes.

2   Account for changes over time, both those that result in loss of a phonemic contrast and/or a decrease in phonetic accuracy and those that establish new phonemic contrasts and/or increase phonetic accuracy.

3   Explain the role of input and account for the relationship between prelinguistic (i.e., babbling) and linguistic development.

4   Account for *phonetic* as well as *phonological* learning and be able to explain the mismatches that often occur between the two.

5   Be consistent with our understanding of speech perception and account for the relationship between perception and production in phonological acquisition.

6   Be compatible with theories of early cognitive and linguistic development and general learning theories.

7   Make testable predictions regarding patterns of acquisition, error types and possible individual differences.

CURRENT THEORIES

In this section, six theories of phonological development are briefly described and their strengths and weaknesses discussed (adapted from Stoel-Gammon and Dunn, 1985). The theories are presented in chronological order beginning with Jakobson's structuralist theory, first published in German in 1941 (English translation, 1968) and ending with Locke's biological theory (1983). It should be noted that there is no consensus as to which 'models' or 'explanations' of phonological development deserve to be called 'theories'. The ones included here were chosen, in part, because they represent a wide range of views and provide diverse sets of claims which can be related to phonological disorders. For more detailed discussions of some of these theories, the reader is referred to Ferguson and Garnica (1975) and Menn (1982).

Structuralist theory. The structuralist theory, proposed by Jakobson in 1941 (English translation, 1968), postulates a relationship between phonological acquisition in children, phonological universals of the languages of the world and phonological dissolution with aphasia. According to the theory, there are two distinct periods of development: babbling and meaningful speech. During the babbling period, the child's productions are 'ephemeral' and include 'an astonishing quantity and diversity of sound productions' that do not adhere to any discernible patterns (Jakobson 1968: 21). With the onset of the second period, meaningful speech, the sound repertoire is severely reduced and speech sounds must be *reacquired* as part of the child's phonemic system. During this period, phonological development follows a universal and innate order of acquisition regulated by a hierarchical set of structural laws. The child begins with two very different sounds, a 'wide' vowel /a/ and a 'forward articulated stop ... generally a labial' (1968: 47). Thereafter, acquisition proceeds in an orderly fashion from 'simple' and undifferentiated to stratified and differentiated'. Although the rate of acquisition may vary from child to child, the relative order of phonemic acquisition is said to be invariant.

Jakobson asserts that acquisition entails the learning of feature contrasts rather than of sounds. The first contrast acquired is *consonantal–vocalic* (/p–a/), followed by the consonantal contrast *nasal–oral* (/p–m/) and then by *grave–acute* (labial–alveolar) (/p–t/). These two consonantal contrasts provide the child with a repertoire of four consonants (/p t m n/) in the early stages of acquisition. For all children, the contrasts that differentiate stops and nasals are said to be acquired before those that differentiate among fricatives, affricates and liquids.

Jakobson's theory has received support from longitudinal case studies (e.g., Velten, 1943; Leopold, 1947; Pacesova, 1968) and larger cross-sectional studies of the acquisition of English (e.g., Templin, 1957; Prather *et al.*, 1975; Stoel-Gammon, 1985). These investigations show that most children acquire the classes of stops and nasals before liquids, fricatives and affricatives. As was predicted for place of articulation, front consonants (i.e., labial, alveolar) are typically acquired before back ones. Although these patterns are common, they are *not* universal either within a given language or across languages.

Studies of acquisition provide support for certain aspects of Jakobson's theory, but there is strong evidence to refute other aspects. First, investigations of the relationship between babbling and meaningful speech (Oller *et al.*, 1976; Vihman *et al.*, 1985) reveal that they are *not* two distinct and independent periods, but, rather, that they share common properties of phonetic repertoire and syllable shapes. Second, the presence of individual variation in the order of phonemic acquisition and in the use of differing 'phonological strategies', does not support the claim that all children adhere to an innate and universal sequence of learning (Stoel-Gammon and Cooper, 1984; Vihman *et al.*, 1985). Finally, Jakobson seems to assume that development proceeds in terms of phonemes and phonemic contrasts from the earliest stages of meaningful speech; however, studies of early word production indicate that, initially, the contrastive unit may be whole words rather than phonemes (Ferguson and Farwell, 1975).

Behaviourist theory. The behaviourist theory, introduced by Mowrer (1952, 1960) and adapted by Winitz (1969) and Olmsted (1966, 1971), emphasizes the role of contingent reinforcement in phonological acquisition and is general enough to account for the speech of 'talking birds' as well as children. According to Mowrer (1952), the following steps are involved:

1 The infant identifies with the caretaker (usually the mother) and attends to her vocalizations during periods of feeding and general nurturing.
2 The infant associates the mother's speech with the primary reinforcements of food and care; as a result, her speech acquires secondary reinforcing properties.
3 The infant's speech-like vocalizations, being similar to the mother's, take on secondary reinforcing values of their own.
4 The infant's productions that most closely resemble adult speech are selectively reinforced by the mother and the infant.

Proceeding through these steps, infant vocalizations are shaped so that they increasingly conform to the speech patterns of the adults in the immediate environment.

Mowrer's theory fulfils some of the requirements listed earlier; specifically, it is compatible with a general theory of learning, behaviour-modification theory, and relates phonological features of meaningful speech to those of babbling. The theory has a major flaw, however, in that it fails to meet the first requirement: it does not account for the data on hand. There is virtually no evidence to support the claim that reinforcement is the primary force in speech-sound acquisition. Deaf infants, unable to hear their own vocalizations or those of their parents, vocalize in spite of a lack of reinforcement. In addition, there is little evidence that mothers selectively reinforce those vocalizations which resemble adult speech. Finally, according to this theory, phonological acquisition involves external shaping of vocal responses in the same way that an animal's responses are shaped through behaviour modification. This view of acquisition as an automatic and mechanistic form of learning is not compatible with studies indicating that children take an active and creative role in learning their sound-system.

Olmsted (1966, 1971) modified Mowrer's theory by incorporating two factors he considered to be important: frequency of phonemes in the adult language and ease of perceptibility of phonemes. In a tightly woven argument based on definitions, postulates, theorems and corollaries, Olmsted (1966) makes three claims: (1) that frequency of occurrence of phones in adult–child speech is roughly the same as in adult–adult speech; (2) that phones which occur frequently in adult–child speech acquire reinforcing properties which increase the likelihood of their use in the child's productions; and (3) that some phones are more discriminable than others and that phones whose articulatory 'components' (e.g., voicing, friction, nasality) are more discriminable are likely to be learned (i.e., produced correctly) earlier than phones whose components are less discriminable.

Using data from a study of perceptual confusion in adults (Miller and Nicely, 1955), Olmsted postulates that in English the components of voicing and nasality are more easily discriminable than friction and duration, which in turn are more discriminable than place of articulation. On the basis of this hierarchy, he then predicts that children will make more errors in place of articulation than friction or duration, more errors in place of articulation, friction and duration than in voicing or nasality, and approximately the same number of errors in voicing the nasality.

Olmsted's model is commendable in that (1) it recognizes the importance of input and perception for an adequate model of phonological development; and (2) it makes testable predictions. In many cases, however, his predictions regarding order of acquisition and frequency of error types have not been supported by empirical studies. Even his own investigation of the development of 100 children failed to support his theory (Olmsted, 1971). In particular, the postulated hierarchy of errors (given above) was not borne out, forcing Olmsted to abandon his assumption that errors and correct predictions would be opposites of each other.

Natural-phonology theory. Stampe's theory of natural phonology centres on the notion of *phonological process*, defined as a mental operation that 'merges a potential phonological opposition into that member of the opposition which least tries the restrictions of the human speech capacity' (Stampe, 1969: 443). Phonological processes are said to be 'natural' because they represent 'natural responses to phonetic forces ... implicit in the human capacity for speech' (Donegan and Stampe, 1979: 130). According to Stampe's theory, children do not actually acquire a phonological system; rather, they begin with a set of innate and universal processes and then learn to suppress or constrain those processes that do not occur in their language. For example, children acquiring English must learn to suppress the process of final-consonant devoicing, because English has both voiced and voiceless obstruents in world-final position, e.g. /s/ and /z/ in *bus* and *buzz*. In contrast, Vietnamese-learning children never need to suppress the devoicing process, because all final obstruents are voiceless in their language.

Researchers in child phonology have adopted Stampe's processes to describe systematic differences in the structural and segmental forms of the child's production when compared with the adult model. Most processes tend to simplify the adult form by deleting sounds or substituting 'easier' sounds for 'harder' ones. Based primarily on studies of English-learning children, four main types of processes have been identified: (1) syllable-structure processes, in which the syllabic shape of a target word is altered; (2) assimilation processes, in which one sound in a word is assimilated to another; (3) substitution processes, in which one class of sounds is substituted for another; and (4) voicing processes, which change the voicing feature. Examples of these processes are provided in Table 1.1.

During the course of phonological acquisition, children constrain processes primarily by suppressing or limiting them. An example of each of these is given below; the form(s) shown in stage 1 represent productions before the process is constrained, and the forms for stage 2 show the changes that occur.

1 Suppression of the process of cluster reduction:

Gloss	Target	Stage 1	Stage 2
blue	[blu]	[bu]	[blu]
green	[grin]	[gin]	[grin]

Table 1.1 Common phonological processes in the speech of normally developing children with examples from English

Process	Examples
Syllable Structure Processes	
Final-consonant deletion	boat [bo]; fish [fɪ]
Unstressed-syllable deletion	tomato ['medo]; elephant ['efənt]
Cluster reduction	snow [no]; brick [bɪk]
Reduplication	water ['wawa]; doggie ['dada]
Epenthesis	big [bɪgə]; blue [bə'lu]
Assimilation Processes	
Velar assimilation	sock [gak]; chicken ['gɪkɪn]
Labial assimilation	sheep [bip]; boat [bop]
Nasal assimilation	bunny ['mʌni]; down [naʊn]
Substitution Processes	
Stopping of fricative and affricates	very ['bɛri]; jaw [da]
Gliding of liquids	rose [woz]; look [jʊk]
Velar fronting	go [do]; cup [tʌp]
Depalatalization[1]	show [so]; chip [tʃɪp]
Voicing Processes	
Prevocalic voicing	pig [bɪg]; happy ['hæbi]
Final devoicing	big [bɪk]; nose [nos]

Note: [1]This process is labelled 'palatal fronting' by some researchers.

2   Limitation of the process of final devoicing so that it applies only to stops:

Gloss	Target	Stage 1	Stage 2
nose	[noz]	[nos]	[noz]
give	[gɪv]	[gɪf]	[gɪv]
mud	[mʌd]	[mʌt]	[mʌt]
bag	[bæg]	[bæk]	[bæk]

Although Stampe's framework has been enthusiastically adopted by many researchers, some important issues remain unresolved. First, there is Stampe's definition of phonological process. Although phonological processes provide a good method for describing error patterns, there is as yet no evidence that they are in fact 'mental operations', as Stampe claims. The problem with this issue (and with the claim itself) is that it is difficult to determine what kind of evidence would support (or refute) the notion of a process as a 'mental operation'.

A second concern is Stampe's view that the child's underlying representation of a word is the same as the adult spoken form. If this were true, the child's perceptual system would have to be fully developed at the onset of meaningful speech. At this point, we do not know enough about children's underlying representations or their perceptual systems to make definitive statements in this regard. As shown below, researchers have differing opinions regarding perception.

Prosodic theory. The prosodic theory, proposed by Waterson (1971, 1981), assumes that speech perception, as well as production, is still developing during the early stages of meaningful speech. According to the theory, children tend to perceive utterances as unanalysed units, rather than as sequences of segments; upon hearing an utterance, they attend to and subsequently attempt to reproduce the most 'salient' features of the utterance. Using a feature set that includes both segmental and suprasegmental features, Waterson (1971) describes utterances in terms of their syllabic structure, stress pattern and segmental characteristics, e.g. continuance, nasality and sibilance. The words *finger, another, window* and *Randall,* for example, are said to share the features of continuance, nasality, non-rounded syllable, voiced ending of all syllables, voiced onset of the second syllable and prominence of the penultimate syllable. Waterson postulated the children perceive the similarities in the structural and segmental patterns of groups of words such as those just cited and reproduce them with an output pattern that duplicates the salient features rather than the specific sounds. Thus, her son produced the words *finger, another, window* and *Randall* with a single basic form ['ɲVɲV] (V = vowel), maintaining the nasality, syllabic structure and stress pattern of the adult forms.

The prosodic theory has several strengths. First, it provides a means for explaining the lack of systematic correspondences between a target phoneme and its pronunciation by the child. If words are perceived in terms of broad features rather than adult-like phonemic units, it is not unexpected that a phoneme will be treated differently in different lexical forms. Second, unlike the theories previously examined, the prosodic theory can account for individual differences in the early stages of acquisition. Third, it considers perception and adult input as important factors of phonological development. The theory is not entirely satisfactory, however, primarily because of its limited scope. It is based on a small corpus from one young child and deals only with the initial stages of acquisition. It does not account for general patterns of acquisition that have been reported, nor does it make predictions regarding error types which might occur.

Cognitive theory. The cognitive theory, developed by Ferguson and his students, is described most completely by Macken and Ferguson (1983; see also Ferguson, 1978). The authors assert that the 'universalist-linguistic' framework adopted by Jakobson (1968) and Stampe (1969, 1973), fails to accommodate two important aspects of phonological development: (1) the presence of individual differences among children acquiring the same language; and (2) longitudinal research showing that acquisition does not proceed in a linear fashion.

In order to account for these phenomena, Macken and Ferguson propose a 'cognitive' model of acquisition based on the premise that children play an *active* role in phonological development by formulating and testing hypotheses regarding the system being acquired. The following are used as evidence to support the model:

1   In the early stages of meaningful speech production, children *selectively* attend to the language addressed to them and choose words with certain phonological characteristics for inclusion in their lexicon while avoiding words with other characteristics.

2   Children are *creative* in acquiring their phonology, as evidenced by the production of phonetic segments and word-like forms not found in the adult language.

3   Children *formulate hypotheses* about the phonological system being acquired and then *test* and *revise* these hypotheses on the basis of linguistic experience.

As evidence of hypothesis formation and hypothesis testing, the authors cite examples of overgeneralization, regression and experimentation that have been observed in individual children.

The cognitive model focuses primarily on the early stages of phonological development, when individual differences are greatest. It postulates that during the initial phases of acquisition children treat words as unanalysed wholes rather than as sequences of segments. As their receptive and productive vocabularies increase, they begin to notice similarities between segments or between sequences of segments, and formulate rules for relating words with similar sounds and/or syllabic shapes. The rules may vary from child to child, and even within a single child there is not always a steady progression towards the adult form, because conflicting rules and competing hypotheses may cause a form to diverge more from the adult model than during the previous stage. Although they focused on individual differences, Macken and Ferguson acknowledge that there are some universal or near-universal patterns in children's speech. They attribute these to the universal nature of the auditory and articulatory systems of children and do not believe that their presence conflicts with their cognitive model of acquisition.

Menn (1976; Kiparsky and Menn, 1977) proposed the 'interactionist–discovery' theory of phonological development, which shares many features with the cognitive theory described here. Phonological acquisition is viewed as a 'problem-solving' activity in which the child plays a central role. Though the two theories are highly similar, with both stressing the child's creativity, Menn pays more attention to the dichotomy between phonetic and phonological learning, hypothesizing that in the early stages words are learned as unanalysable *phonetic* forms. Subsequently, these words are segmented and reorganized on the basis of phonemes.

Like Waterson's prosodic theory, the cognitive theory can easily account for individual differences in early development. It goes further than the prosodic theory in providing explanations for phenomena not considered in most other theories, e.g. lexical selection, regression, the use of phonological strategies, etc. Although its coverage of the early stages of development is excellent, it pays little attention to other, equally important issues, e.g. (1) later development; (2) the relationship of perception and production; and (3) the similarities (general patterns) observed in studies of large groups of subjects. In addition, it fails to make testable predictions regarding phonological development.

Biological theory. Locke (1980, 1983) proposes a model of phonological acquisition that emphasizes the similarities between the phonological patterns of late babbling and those of early meaningful speech. The model has three basic premises:

1 The prelinguistic vocalizations of infants from all linguistic environments are highly similar; during the late babbling period, stops, nasals and glides account for more than 90 per cent of the consonantal phones, whereas fricatives, affricates and liquids are infrequent.
2 The phonetic repertoire and phonological patterns of early meaningful speech resemble closely those of the late babbling period, with both dominated by stops, nasals and glides; because the babbling patterns are universal, so are the patterns of the first words.
3 Frequently occurring sounds from the babbling repertoire (i.e.,

stops, nasals, glides) serve as substitutes for infrequent babbling sounds (i.e., fricatives, affricates, liquids). The exact substitution patterns depend on perceptual similarity between frequent and infrequent segments. Using data on adult perceptual confusions (Wang and Bilger, 1973) Locke predicts, for example, that [b] would substitute for /v/ and [d] for/ð/.

According to the model, there are three major stages of phonological acquisition. During the prelinguistic stage, infants come to realize that their vocalizations are capable of conveying information regarding basic needs or desires; their productions can be recognized as requests, calls, etc. Proto-words (i.e., word-like forms not based on an adult model) may appear towards the end of this stage.

The second stage begins when the child attempts to produce conventional words. Phonetically, these productions are much like those of the previous stage; phonologically they are different. Meaningful speech, unlike babbling, involves cognitive processes such as recognition of adult forms, storage and retrieval of words and pattern matching, which were not needed in babbling. The third stage is characterized by marked changes in the child's phonological system. The sounds and sound patterns of meaningful speech no longer resemble those of babbling and become increasingly similar to those of the adult phonological system being acquired. During this stage vocabulary increases rapidly and the child begins to produce words with increasing phonological complexity. As the system develops, phonological acquisition ceases to be dominated solely by phonetic (or biological) tendencies. Instead, an interaction of phonetic and cognitive factors allows the possibility of individual differences in the course of development.

The strengths of Locke's theory are that it (1) relates the phonological development of the prelinguistic and linguistic periods; (2) provides a partial explanation of the relationship between perception and production; (3) accounts for the similar developmental processes observed across children from different linguistic environments; and (4) attempts to relate the phonetic and cognitive components of acquisition.

Weaknesses of this theory can be attributed, in part, to the emphasis given to universal or near-universal patterns of development. Little attention is given to studies showing early individual differences in acquisition and the use of phonological strategies in the early stages is not discussed. Here again, as in some of the previously cited theories, it seems to be assumed that in the early stages the child's role in phonological acquisition is relatively passive.

Comparison of current theories

The theories discussed above can be divided into two groups on the basis of their views of the child's role in acquiring the phonological system. The first group, comprised of the theories of Jakobson, Stampe, Locke, Mowrer and Olmsted, asserts that the critical factors in acquisition are largely predetermined or external; consequently, the child plays a relatively passive role. According to the theories in the second group, comprised of Waterson, Menn and Macken and Ferguson, children play an active role in phonological development.

In the first group, Jakobson (structuralist theory) asserts that a set of innate and universal 'laws of irreversible solidarity' governs the order of acquisition of distinctive feature contrasts; Stampe (natural-phonology theory) posits that phonological processes, reflecting the natural limitations of human vocal production and perception, are the primary determinants of phonological development; and Locke (biological theory) argues that universal babbling patterns are the crucial elements in phonological acquisition during the period of meaningful speech. Mowrer (behaviourist theory) emphasizes the role of contingent reinforcement and selective shaping of the child's productions by the adult and Olmsted adds frequency of occurrence of a sound and perceptual confusions to Mowrer's notion of reinforcement. Although these theories differ as to the specific factors critical to phonological acquisition, they are in agreement that these factors are either external (e.g. adult reinforcement) or predetermined (e.g. the innate set of phonological processes) and consequently the child's role in acquiring the phonological system is relatively passive.

In contrast, the theories of Waterson (prosodic theory), Menn and Macken and Ferguson (cognitive theory) view phonological acquisition as a problem-solving activity in which the child plays an active role. The child is seen as using a variety of strategies to master the tasks involved in learning accurately to perceive and produce the sounds of his or her language. Evidence for the problem-solving approach includes selectivity in early word choice and individual differences in phonological patterns of early meaningful speech.

CHARACTERISTICS OF DISORDERED PHONOLOGY

Before attempting to relate the theories of phonological development described above to phonological disorders, a brief description of the characteristics of disordered phonology and the differences between normal and disordered phonological development is needed. To date, published studies of developmental phonological disorders have focused almost exclusively on young British and American children, thereby precluding the possibility of making firm statements regarding universal patterns. Thus, the following list of characteristics commonly found in the phonologies of children identified as being disordered (from Stoel-Gammon and Dunn, 1985; Grunwell, 1987) must be regarded as preliminary until supported by cross-linguistic research. The list contains six characteristics, some of which are inter-related. It is unlikely that a particular child will evidence all of them; in most cases, three or four features will co-occur in the system of a phonologically disordered subject. The first two characteristics are derived from analysis of the child's system *independent* of the adult system; the others are based on a *relational analysis* comparing the child's system with that of the adult.

1 *Restricted set of speech sounds.* In many cases, a child of three to four years may produce only stop, nasal and glide consonants and a limited set of vowels. Such a repertoire often occurs in the *very* young normally developing child, but by age two, a majority of children produce words with some fricative or liquid phones (Stoel-Gammon, 1985).

2 *Limited word and syllable shapes.* The most typical constraints on syllable structure are lack of consonant clusters and lack of final consonants leaving V (vowel) and CV (consonant–vowel) as the predominant syllable types. Bisyllabic words are usually CVCV forms and in some cases only reduplicated syllables will appear (e.g. [wawa]). Again, these patterns typify the productions of very young children but more diverse word and syllable shapes typically occur by the age of two or shortly thereafter.

3 *Persistence of error patterns.* In normally developing children, the frequency of occurrence of many phonological processes (see Table 1.1, above) declines rapidly so that by age three, the processes of final-consonant deletion, reduplication, velar fronting, unstressed-syllable deletion, prevocalic voicing and labial, velar and nasal assimi-lation are rare in the speech of English-acquiring subjects. Among phonologically disordered children, however, these error types often persist well beyond the age-appropriate levels.

4 *Chronological mismatch.* For normal children, there is a fairly regular sequence for the disappearance of error types (see Grunwell, 1981); some children with disordered phonology, however, fail to conform to the normal timetable, thereby creating a phonological

system which is advanced in some respects but severely delayed in others. An example of this sort of 'chronological mismatch' is a child who produces a full range of clusters in initial position while having no final consonants.

5 *Unusual error types.* A number of error types observed in the speech of phonologically disordered children occur rarely or for only brief periods in the normal child. Error patterns in this class include atypical substitution or deletion patterns (e.g. initial-consonant deletion, glottal substitutions), persistent vowel errors, the creation of word patterns and the use of suprasegmental features to mark segmental information. Cross-linguistic studies of normal and disordered phonological development may show that these error patterns are atypical for English but normal for other languages. This topic clearly needs further research.

6 *Extensive variability, but lack of progress.* All children show some degree of variability at both the word and phoneme level during the period of phonological acquisition. In normally developing subjects, this phenomenon is typically associated with phonological advance as the system is reorganized, or with improvement in accuracy as older incorrect forms vary with newer more correct ones. Among phonologically disordered children, variability often occurs without any apparent advance at the phonetic or phonological levels; in these cases, variability seems to be an inherent feature of the children's phonological systems.

THE RELATIONSHIP BETWEEN PHONOLOGICAL DISORDERS AND THEORIES OF PHONOLOGICAL DEVELOPMENT

This section discusses the theories of phonological acquisition described on pages 18–27 in light of the characteristics of disordered phonology outlined above. Although none of the proposed theories specifically addresses the issue of atypical patterns of development, each would lend itself to a set of assumptions regarding disordered phonologies.

The first three features described in the previous section (restricted set of speech sounds, limited word and syllable shapes and persistence of error patterns) indicate that disordered phonological systems tend to plateau at an early level of development, failing to progress towards the adult language. These characteristics typically create a sound system composed of a small repertoire of consonants, usually stops, nasals and glides, and syllable shapes limited to single vowels or simple consonant–vowel combinations. The resultant system could be considered normal for a child under two years with a vocabulary of 200–300 words, but not for a three- or four-year-old with a vocabulary of 1,000 words or more.

The 'immature' productions of the phonologically disordered child can be accounted for, in part, by the theories of Jakobson, Stampe and Locke, although each provides a different explanation. The sound and syllable types of phonologically disordered subjects conform to Jakobson's claim that acquisition is governed by a universal set of 'laws of irreversible solidarity'; the developmental sequence described by Jakobson is maintained, but the child moves at a much slower rate in learning the features associated with phonemic contrasts and fails to progress beyond the earliest levels of development. Stampe's set of *phonological processes* can also account for a limited phonetic repertoire and simple syllable types characteristic of a phonologically disordered child; here again, it would be argued that the pattern of development is normal, but the rate of development is atypical. Finally, Locke's biological theory predicts a preponderance of stops, nasals and glides and consonant–vowel syllables in early meaningful speech, the exact pattern seen in many phonologically disordered subjects (Dinnsen and Chin, 1988); disorders associated with such a repertoire would presumably be viewed as 'delayed' but not necessarily 'deviant'.

Although each of the theories cited above can accommodate the first three characteristics identified in the previous section, none provides a possible explanation for the arrested development which occurs. Moreover, it would be difficult for these theories to account for the last three characteristics in the list: chronological mismatch, unusual error patterns and extensive variability. Chronological mismatch would create a phonological system which fails to conform to Jakobson's predetermined order of acquisition of sounds and features, and unusual error patterns would fall outside Stampe's set of 'natural phonological processes' and Locke's predictions on the nature of errors in child speech.

The cognitive theories of Waterson, Menn, and Macken and Ferguson can account for these phenomena by postulating that phonologically disordered children form unusual hypotheses regarding the phonological patterns of their mother tongue. Implementation of these hypotheses would then result in an atypical phonological system. The characteristic of extensive variability might be explained as a consequence of competing hypotheses applied in a variety of orders. Thus, the strength of the cognitively based models is that they can accommodate extensive individual variation in phonological development. Their major weakness is that they fail to predict the extent to which the sound systems of many phonologically disordered subjects resemble the systems of younger normal children.

In contrast to the deterministic and cognitive theories cited above, Mowrer's behaviourist model does not appear to be capable of accounting for any of the characteristics of disordered phonological systems. Since contingent reinforcement is viewed as the critical feature in this theory, one would have to hypothesize that lack of reinforcement was a causal factor associated with phonological disorders. To date, there is no evidence to support this view, but it is possible that a phonological disorder could affect adult input. If a child's speech is highly unintelligible, it is likely that the amount and complexity of adult speech to that child will be reduced, thereby creating a form of input which is qualitatively and quantitatively different from that of a normally developing peer.

In summary, each theory, except perhaps Mowrer's, can account reasonably well for some aspects of phonological disorders, but none can easily handle all of the data on hand. The inadequacies are due in large part to the fact that current theories tend to focus on a particular aspect of the developing phonological system, for example, on the order of acquisition of speech sounds, on error types or on individual differences. A theory which can account for phonological disorders would have to be more comprehensive, and would of necessity pay attention to the mechanisms involved in speech and hearing as well as to patterns of individual differences and general trends. Suggestions for such a theory are provided in the section which follows.

TOWARDS A BROADER MODEL: SOME SUGGESTIONS

A major shortcoming of current theories is that they tend to emphasize either common patterns or individual differences, when in fact both are present and must be accounted for. Most theories tend to equate biology with similarities and cognition with individual differences. We must, however, be wary of oversimplifying the possible ways in which biological and cognitive bases of phonological development are reflected in patterns of similarity and differences across children. As Locke (1988) pointed out, children can differ in the anatomical and neural features that underlie their speech-production mechanisms; consequently, one cannot assume that interchild

variations (individual differences) result solely from cognitive differences. Further, variation in cognitive style (i.e., analytic vs gestalt
approach to language learning) may be genetically based. Thus, a
theory which can explain common patterns as well as individual
differences must incorporate both biological and cognitive aspects of
development.

These considerations suggest that we need a broader model than
those currently proposed, one which includes at least three major
components: auditory-perceptual, cognitive-linguistic and neuromotor-articulatory. The cognitive-linguistic component is responsible
for recognizing and storing word forms, for constructing and testing
rules of output, and for comparing input to output. For the most part,
current theories focus on this component, with minimal attention
given to the role of the speech and hearing mechanisms or to the
effects of abnormalities in these mechanisms. However, these
mechanisms, which are reflected in the other two components of the
proposed model, are an essential part of any theory of phonological
disorders because they allow us to see the interactions between structure and function in the developing system.

The auditory-perceptual component is responsible for the ability to
attend to and perceive linguistic input. For normally developing
children, this component allows for the discrimination and categorization of speech sounds according to the patterns of the mother
tongue. In the disordered population, a deficit in the auditory system,
as with a hearing-impaired child, has a profound effect on the
development of phonological system and on the phonetic features of
speech production. To complicate matters, it is increasingly clear that
an understanding of the nature of a disorder must incorporate not
only the current state of the auditory system, but its history as well.
For example, a child with recurrent otitis media (inflammation in the
middle ear cavity) from nine to twenty-four months may evidence a
phonological disorder at the age of three. Although his or her hearing
status may be normal at this age, the disorder may be attributed to a
fluctuating hearing loss during the first two years of life. The impact
of such a loss could also negatively influence the child's ability to
categorize speech sounds.

The neuromotor-articulatory component is responsible for
planning and executing articulatory gestures associated with speech
production. Although some would argue that abnormalities of the
oral-motor mechanism would adversely affect only the surface
phonetics, leaving the underlying phonological system intact, here
again, we must consider not only the present state but past experience

as well. For example, a child with ankyloglossia (tongue tie) may have problems producing lingual sounds even after the frenulum has been clipped and normal function has been restored to the tongue. Thus, problems which appear 'phonological' in nature, with no observable physical cause, may in fact stem from earlier abnormalities.

Finally, a broader theory should include some discussion of the role of maturation in phonological development. As pointed out in a previous section, the sound systems of some of phonologically disordered children appear to result from arrested development. The system is not aberrant when considered in isolation, but is clearly not normal when age or lexicon size is taken into consideration. It is as though the child is working with an immature system which is not yet ready to move on to the next developmental stage. Whether this immaturity is biologically based remains to be determined. In any event, the notion of 'readiness' or maturity is an additional parameter which needs to be considered.

CONCLUSION

This chapter has reviewed current theories of phonological development, showing that they can be divided into two groups based on their views of the child's role in phonological acquisition. One group focuses on common patterns, asserting that children are relatively passive in the acquisition process and that development is largely innate or is guided by external factors such as contingent reinforcement or input frequency. The other group focuses on individual differences, arguing that the presence of these differences shows that children play an active role in learning their sound system.

When the theories were evaluated in light of our knowledge of phonological disorders, it was found that each was able to account for *some* aspects of disordered phonology, but that none was entirely successful, primarily because each tended to focus either on common patterns or on individual differences. Suggestions for a more comprehensive model, one which would incorporate both biological and cognitive aspects, were then presented. It was argued that an explanation of phonological disorders must also include consideration of both the past and present state of a child's auditory and articulatory system. The proposals outlined in the previous section are not intended as specific answers to specific questions, but as a general construct to be used as a framework for future theories of phonological development.

ACKNOWLEDGEMENT

Preparation of this chapter was supported in part by a grant from the National Institutes of Health (NS 26521-01). The author would like to thank Judith Stone for her comments on an earlier draft.

REFERENCES

Dinnsen, D. and Chin, S. (1988) 'Some phonological constraints on functional speech disorders', paper presented at the annual meeting of the American Speech–Language–Hearing Association, Boston, MA.

Donegan, P. and Stampe, D. (1979) 'The study of natural phonology', in D. Dinnsen (ed.) *Current Approaches to Phonological Theory*, Bloomington: Indiana University Press, 126–73.

Ferguson, C.A. (1978) 'Learning to pronounce: the earliest stages of phonological development in the child', in F.D. Minifie and L.L. Lloyd (eds) *Communicative and Cognitive Abilities – Early Behavioral Assessment*, Baltimore: University Park Press, pp. 273–97.

Ferguson, C.A. and Farwell, C. (1975) 'Words and sounds in early language acquisition: English initial consonants in the first fifty words', *Language* 51: 419–39.

Ferguson, C.A. and Garnica, O. (1975) 'Theories of phonological development', in E. Lenneberg and E. Lenneberg (eds) *Foundations of Language Development*, vol. 1, New York: Academic Press, pp. 149–80.

Grunwell, P. (1981) *The Nature of Phonological Disability in Children*, New York: Academic Press.

Grunwell, P. (1987) 'Evaluation and explanation of developmental phonological disorders', paper presented at the First International Symposium on Specific Speech and Language Disorders in Children, Reading, England.

Jakobson, R. (1968) *Child Language, Aphasia, and Phonological Universals* (A.R. Keiler, trans.), The Hague: Mouton. (Original work published 1941.)

Kiparsky, P. and Menn, L. (1977) 'On the acquisition of phonology', in J. Macnamara (ed.) *Language Learning and Thought*, New York: Academic Press, pp. 47–78.

Leopold, W.F. (1947) *Speech Development of a Bilingual Child: A Linguist's Record*, vol. II: *Sound Learning in the First Two Years*, Evanston, Il: Northwestern University.

Locke, J. (1980), 'The prediction of child speech errors: implications for a theory of acquisition', in G. Yeni-Komshian, J.F. Kavanagh and C.A. Ferguson (eds) *Child Phonology*, vol. 1, New York: Academic Press, pp. 193–209.

Locke, J. (1983) *Phonological Acquisition and Change*, New York: Academic Press.

Locke, J. (1988) 'Variation in human biology and child phonology: a response to Good and Ingram', *Journal of Child Language* 15: 663–8.

Macken, M. and Ferguson, C. (1983) 'Cognitive aspects of phonological development: model, evidence and issues', in K.E. Nelson (ed.) *Children's Language*, vol. 4, New York: Gardner Press, pp. 256–82.

Menn, L. (1976) 'Evidence for an interactionist–discovery theory of child phonology', *Papers and Reports on Child Language Development* 12: 169–77.

Menn, L. (1982) 'Theories of phonological development', *Annals of the New York Academy of Science* 379: 130–7.

Miller, G.A. and Nicely, P.E. (1955) 'An analysis of perceptual confusions among some English consonants', *Journal of the Acoustical Society of America* 27: 338–52.

Mowrer, O.H. (1952) 'Speech development in the young child: the autism theory of speech development and some clinical applications', *Journal of Speech and Hearing Disorders* 17: 263–8.

Mowrer, O.H. (1960) *Learning Theory and Symbolic Processes*, New York: Wiley.

Oller, D.K., Wieman, L.A., Doyle, W.J. and Ross, C. (1976) 'Infant babbling and speech', *Journal of Child Language* 3: 1–11.

Olmsted, D. (1966) 'A theory of the child's learning of phonology', *Language* 42: 531–5.

Olmsted, D. (1971) *Out of the Mouth of Babes*, The Hague: Mouton.

Pacesova, J. (1968) *The Development of Vocabulary in the Child*, Brno: University J.E. Purkyne.

Prather, E., Hedrick, D. and Kern, C. (1975) 'Articulation development in children aged two to four years', *Journal of Speech and Hearing Disorders* 40: 179–91.

Shriberg, L. (1982), 'Diagnostic assessment of developmental phonological disorders', in M. Crary (ed.) *Phonological Intervention*, San Diego: College-Hill Press, pp. 35–60.

Stampe, D. (1969) 'The acquisition of phonetic representation', *Papers from the Fifth Regional Meeting of the Chicago Linguistic Society*, Chicago: Chicago Linguistic Society, 433–44.

Stampe, D. (1973) 'A dissertation on natural phonology', unpublished doctoral dissertation, University of Chicago.

Stoel-Gammon, C. (1985) 'Phonetic inventories, 15–24 months: a longitudinal study', *Journal of Speech and Hearing Research* 28: 505–12.

Stoel-Gammon, C. and Cooper, J. (1984) 'Patterns of early lexical and phonological development', *Journal of Child Language* 11: 247–71.

Stoel-Gammon, C. and Dunn, C. (1985) *Normal and Disordered Phonology in Children*, Austin, TX: Pro-Ed.

Templin, M.C. (1957) *Certain Language Skills in Children: their Development and Interrelationships* (Institute of Child Welfare Monographs 26), Minneapolis: University of Minnesota Press.

Velten, H.V. (1943) 'The growth of phonemic and lexical patterns in infant language', *Language* 19: 281–92.

Vihman, M., Macken, M.A., Miller, R., Simmons, H. and Miller, J. (1985) 'From babbling to speech: a reassessment of the continuity issue', *Language* 61: 397–445.

Wang, M.D. and Bilger, R.C. (1973) 'Consonant confusions in noise: a study of perceptual features', *Journal of Acoustical Society of America* 54: 248–66.

Waterson, N. (1971) 'Child phonology: a prosodic view', *Journal of Linguistics* 7: 179–211.

Waterson, N. (1981) 'A tentative developmental model of phonological representation', in T. Myers, J. Laver and J. Anderson (eds) *The Cognitive Representation of Speech*, Amsterdam: North Holland, pp. 323–33.

Winitz, H. (1969) *Articulatory Acquisition and Behavior*, Englewood Cliffs, N.J.: Prentice Hall.

2 Developmental phonological disorders from a clinical-linguistic perspective

Pamela Grunwell

When children fail to communicate because their speech cannot be understood we need to address the question of *why* their pronunciation is inadequate from three points of view. First, from an adult viewpoint we need to identify why it is difficult to understand the speech of any particular child: i.e., in what ways are the pronunciation patterns different from the normal adult (target) pronunciation patterns? Second, from the developmental viewpoint we need to investigate why the speech of any particular child is judged to be unacceptable and/or inadequate by comparison with that of his or her peers: i.e., in what ways are the pronunciation patterns different from those expected of children developing normally? Finally, from a clinical viewpoint (though of course the two preceding questions also have a clinical motivation), we need to explain why any particular child is experiencing difficulties in learning to pronounce: i.e. in what ways can the disordered development of pronunciation patterns be related to identifiable differences and/or deficiencies in the prerequisite abilities and potential of the child?

In attempting to answer these questions and therefore in seeking to understand the nature of the difficulties experienced by children with developmental phonological disorders we need to apprehend the nature of spoken language, both normal and disordered, and the nature of the development of spoken language, again both normal and disordered. It will be evident, therefore, that a knowledge of procedures for phonetic and phonological analysis is required, as is also a description of the process and patterns of speech development. Clinical phonological assessments apply these two information bases in the descriptive evaluation of children's pronunciation patterns and provide direct and detailed answers to the first two questions delineated above. What is less readily appreciated is that phonological descriptions also have a contribution to make to the clinical evaluation of the nature of a child's speech disorder; i.e., they provide information which must be taken into account in formulating an answer to the third question.

In this chapter we shall be considering the fundamental concepts that are required to provide answers to all three of these questions in the context of developmental phonological disorders. We shall then consider the characteristics of children with these disorders, both from the clinical and linguistic perspectives. Having established a common frame of reference we shall then consider selected issues in the clinical management of children with these disorders: specifically, the construction and relevance of selected assessment procedures and the conceptualization and identification of treatment goals implied by and derived from the phonological approach to assessment and evaluation.

In describing the nature of speech disorders it is essential that we are aware of the fundamental theoretical distinction between a phonetic and a phonological analysis. From a phonetic analysis we build up a detailed description of the auditory, acoustic and articu- latory characteristics of speech from the physical and physiological perspectives. Such a description provides important information, in the instance of children with speech disorders, about the abilities, potential and constraints of the child's speech-production mechanism. But this type of description does not provide any inform- ation about how these phonetic resources are being employed in communication through spoken language. Phonology (or functional phonetics, as it has sometimes been termed) describes the organiz- ation and functions of the phonetic constituents of speech as the signalling system of spoken language. A phonological analysis of the speech of a child with a speech disorder is therefore important in that it provides a description of the *patterns* of pronunciation used in the child's own spoken language, and by comparison with the expected (adult) patterns, it identifies the communicative implications of the speech disorder. That is, it describes the functional consequences of the disordered pronunciation patterns which are manifested by failures to signal the sound differences required to communicate meaning differences.

The theoretical distinction between phonetics and phonology has been of critical significance in the evolution of our understanding of developmental phonological disorders. As we shall see in the second section below, children with these pronunciation problems do not appear to have any identifiable physical or physiological disabilities that would handicap their learning to pronounce. Yet they are evidently experiencing major difficulties in this aspect of language development. It has therefore been proposed (e.g. by Ingram, 1976; Grunwell, 1981; Stoel-Gammon and Dunn, 1985), that these children's speech problems can be viewed as *phonological* learning disorders. This breakthrough in our conceptualization of the nature of the children's pronunciation problems stimulated an upsurge of research using phonological analysis procedures, which in turn led to new insights into these disorders.

One important recent development which is in part attributable to the research findings of studies of developmental phonological disorders (as well as studies of different types of acquired speech disorders) is the proposal that a two-way distinction between phonetics and phonology is too simplistic as a model of speech production, and therefore as the basis for identifying the components involved in pronunciation development and disorders. Hewlett (1985), for example, proposes a model that has three components:

1 *phonology:* the highest stage in terms of cortical functioning, when the words to be spoken are selected, together with their phonological representation in terms of a stored image of their phonological constituents; i.e. this is the cognitive level.
2 *phonetics:* the intermediate stage at which the phonological constituents are converted into the movement sequences for pronunciation; this stage therefore involves selection, ordering and sequencing of stored motor patterns; i.e. this is the organizational level of motor control and co-ordination.
3 *articulation:* the peripheral stage in speech production when the articulators produce the movements which create the speech sounds; i.e. this is the only directly observable level of speech production.

This three-way distinction has considerable potential in providing insights into the normal development of spoken language and both disordered development and disordered speech *per se*. It will be evident therefore that this model is particularly valuable, especially as it provides a common framework for addressing all three questions posed at the beginning of this chapter.

It should be noted that the manner in which this descriptive model is presented and employed in clinical descriptions and evaluations is different from the way the two-term distinction between phonetics and phonology was routinely applied. The latter has typically been used to describe the characteristic differences in the *data* of child speech and speech disorders (see, for example, Grunwell 1987). The new three-term distinction has been specifically proposed as a *model* of the speech-production process. This shift in orientation is high-lighted by both Hewlett (1985) and Grunwell (1985a) in respect to its implications for the clinician:

> In speech pathology it is now quite common to distinguish between 'phonetic' or 'articulatory' disorders and 'phonological' disorders. This is one of the fruits of the application of linguistics to speech pathology, and it allows pathologies in which speech sounds are affected to be differentiated according to whether the abnormality is associated with the speech production mechanism itself or whether it has something to do with the way in which speech sounds function in distinguishing one word from another in the speaker's native language. The basic distinction is obviously a useful one. But it will be argued that linguistics has provided a model which is inappropriately for speech pathology 'data-oriented' rather than 'speaker-oriented' and that this has led to confusion, to an over-simplification of the distinction and to a lack of consideration of the possible effects of phonetic factors upon the phonological level, especially in the context of language development.
>
> (Hewlett, 1985: 155–6)

Grunwell (1985a), however, suggests that the two types of approaches to an analysis identified by Hewlett should remain available at least in principle. A phonetic and phonological analysis of spoken language provides a systematic description of the patterns observed in a sample of a person's speech output. It can also be interpreted as a psycholinguistic explanation of the process involved in the person's production of the speech sample and the patterns therein. These are the two viewpoints that Hewlett termed 'data-oriented' versus 'speaker-oriented'. The clinician can elect to view their analyses either as descriptions or explanations.

While one would not wish to restrict the clinician's freedom to choose a descriptive or explanatory interpretation, it is clearly the explanatory approach that will lead in the longer term to clinically applicable insights into the nature of speech disorders and disordered speech development. Indeed, Stoel-Gammon and Dunn (1985: 203), at the very end of their book, signpost this approach as the way forward for studies of developmental phonological disorders:

> We join others in the field ... in stressing the need for investigations directed towards explaining rather than describing phono-

logical development and disorders. Descriptions are, of course an important part of research in these areas, but they are only a first step. They must be complemented by studies and theories aimed at explaining the phenomena that have been described.

We shall return to a discussion of possible explanations of these disorders at the end of the next section.

THE CHARACTERISTICS OF DEVELOPMENTAL PHONOLOGICAL DISORDERS

In considering the characteristics of these disorders we shall first of all identify the clinical population, i.e. the presenting characteristics of the children with these speech problems, and then we shall describe and discuss the characteristics of their speech.

An appreciable proportion of children who are identified as having language-learning difficulties exhibit specific pronunciation problems that appear to inhibit their development of spoken language. For some of these children their language-learning difficulties appear to be restricted to the learning of the pronunciation patterns of their language. They appear to be potentially capable of producing lengthy utterances which are apparently grammatically structured and appropriate to the context in which they occur. Their vocabulary appears to be quite extensive and they evidence an adequate ability to comprehend spoken language. Yet in contrast to these apparently well-developed linguistic abilities, their speech is virtually unintelligible. There is, however, no detectable organic pathology which would account for their pronunciation difficulties. These children's speech is unintelligible primarily as a result of consonantal deviations. Their problems can be confidently diagnosed at 4;0; prior to this age many children are often difficult to understand. By approximately 4;0–4;6 the phonological system has largely been acquired by children developing spoken language normally; only a few aspects of the segmental phonology remain to be mastered, though considerable articulatory maturation occurs after this age (Grunwell, 1986). There is no organic base to these children's speech problems: they have normal hearing for speech, no anatomical or physiological abnormalities, nor any detectable neurological dysfunction relevant to speech production. They also appear capable of learning, with adequate intellectual abilities and an appropriate psychosocial environment.

These are the characteristics of children with a *specific* phonological disorder. In many instances these children exhibit delay in the development of other aspects of the production of spoken language, especially in syntax and morphology, but also quite often in vocabulary too. These linguistic difficulties may be indicative of a general language-learning disability, in which instance the phonological disorder is not in fact 'specific', but is part of the overall problem (see, for example, Schwartz *et al.*, 1980; for a brief review of this issue see Grunwell, 1986). There are, however, some children (it may be only a small minority) for whom the primary learning difficulty is phonological and the grammatical problems are derivative from, and secondary to, the primary phonological disorder. These secondary grammatical difficulties may result from the presence of the phonological problem, as a consequence of two types of behaviour patterns induced by the child's repeated failure to make himself understood. First, the child himself may restrict his output in terms of utterance length and complexity and in regard to the selection of vocabulary items, in an attempt to improve his chances of being understood. Second, because the child cannot be understood by the adults with whom he interacts, they in their turn are not able to converse effectively with the child and are thus unable to provide the feedback and facilitative types of responses which children usually receive from adults. Therefore the child's language development may be hindered. Thus, while there is a small clinical population with very specific phonological disabilities, the vast majority of language-disordered children exhibit both grammatical and phonological learning difficulties.

The defining characteristics of developmental phonological disorders explicitly exclude the identifiable presence of any organic pathology affecting the child's speech-production system which might therefore be regarded as the 'cause' of the pronunciation problems. This is an essential exclusion if we are to draw the distinction between disorders of phonological learning, knowledge and organization and disorders of articulatory production. However, once this distinction has been clearly appreciated we can reconsider the nature of disordered articulatory production in children. Given that children with organic pathologies, for example cleft palate, also have to develop their pronunciation systems, it is feasible that some of these children will experience difficulties with the learning process that are not attributable to the organic pathology. This possibility needs to be borne in mind when investigating the nature of the pronunciation patterns and the associated underlying problems of such children. Therefore a phonological assessment is required in such instances as well as phonetically based investigations (Grunwell, 1987a, d; Grunwell and Russell, 1987).

To return to the characteristics of children with specific phonological disorders with no identifiable organic pathology, we need now
to consider the characteristics of their speech and spoken language.
Grunwell (1981), after an extensive review of the literature to that
date, summarized the phonetic characteristics as follows:

1   The number and variety of different phonetic segments are
    restricted.
2   The range of phonetic feature combinations is restricted, though
    some types of segments occur that do not occur in the speech of
    normal speakers. Certain common restrictions are noted:
    (a) it is often the case that the number of places of articulation is
        restricted and/or there is a predominance of one place of
        articulation;
    (b) fricatives rarely occur at more than one, maximally two,
        places of articulation and are used infrequently;
    (c) affricates are frequently absent;
    (d) there is usually only one non-nasal sonorant;
    (e) the voiced/voiceless distinction between obstruents is often
        lacking.
3   The phonotactic structures of syllables tend towards CVCV. As a
    result of this tendency:
    (a) there are few if any consonant clusters at any position in
        syllable and word structure;
    (b) there is a tendency towards open syllables;
    (c) the only articulated consonants that occur with any
        frequency in syllable-final positions (both within word and
        word-final) are nasals, although the occurrence of a word-
        final fricative is occasionally noted;
    (d) the glottal stop has a high frequency of occurrence, especially
        in word-final and syllable-initial within word positions.
        (NB: these are the phonetic characteristics of children
        learning English who have development phonological disor-
        ders.)

These phonetic characteristics point to an extremely restricted phonetic inventory and a restricted range of distributional possibilities.
From this it can be inferred that the children's phonological systems
will also be restricted with the inevitable consequence already high-
lighted, that the children's speech will be virtually unintelligible.

On the basis of a strictly autonomous analysis of the child's phonological system as an independent phonology, Grunwell (1981, 1985b)
defined the following phonological (or 'systemic') characteristics:

1   The children's phonologies are communicatively inadequate to the requirements of their grammatical and lexical systems to signal meaning differences. This results from major restrictions in the number of contrasts the children's phonologies are capable of encoding both segmentally and phonotactically.

2   The children's phonologies tend not to exploit their contrastive potential by employing all the possible (and necessary) combinations of features. They are therefore phonologically asymmetrical and uneconomical in their use of potential feature contrasts.

3   The children's phonologies are variable in their realizations of words and in their mapping on to the target phonological system. This entails lack of predictability in the phonological patterns and therefore uncertainty for the listener as to the meanings being communicated.

4   In developing phonologies, however, there must be some variability as this is the precursor to change. Children with phonological disorders fail to make changes spontaneously: they have static variable systems.

These phonological characteristics taken together with the phonetic characteristics pinpoint the aspects of the children's pronunciation patterns that are usually different from the adult pronunciation patterns and which account for the inability on the part of the adult listeners to understand the children's speech. In the descriptive assessment of any particular child the analytical procedures will identify precisely where the communicative inadequacies of the child's pronunciation system occur and therefore provide the answer to the first of the three questions posed above.

In considering the characteristics of the child's phonological system, we have already made reference to the developmental dimension of the disorder in regard to the occurrence of non-progressive variability. In fact, the developmental characteristics of these disorders are the best attested of the three types of characteristics. Furthermore, they have been found to have cross-linguistic relevance. They also provide the basis for the most popular approach to the evaluation of these disorders, as they are themselves based on descriptive assessment procedures employing phonological-process analysis (see further below). The developmental characteristics of children's phonological disorders are as follows:

1   *Persisting normal processes* are those normal phonological simplifying processes which remain in the child's pronunciation

patterns long after the age at which they would be expected to have been suppressed. If the processes evidenced in a data sample are all normal and are homogeneous in terms of their chronology, then it is clear that a child's phonological development is delayed to a greater or lesser extent, depending upon his or her age, or is 'arrested' at a particular stage of development.

2   *Chronological mismatch* is the co-occurrence of some of the earliest normal simplifying processes with some patterns of pronunciation characteristic of later stages in phonological development. Such uneven progress by comparison with the normal chronology of development is clearly suggestive of disrupted or disordered development.

3   *Unusual/idiosyncratic processes* are simplifying patterns which have been rarely attested in normal development or which appear to be different from normal developmental processes and which may therefore be idiosyncratic. Leonard (1985) classifies these unusual phonological behaviours into two categories: (a) salient sound changes with readily detectable systematicity, e.g. early sound replaced by late sounds, additions to adult surface forms, use of sounds absent from the target language or from natural languages; (b) salient sound changes with less readily detectable systematicity, e.g. context-based speech patterns such as harmony/assimilation, dissimilation, metathesis.

4   *Variable use of processes* occurs where more than one simplifying process routinely operates with the same target type of structures, so that the child's realizations of these target types are variable and unpredictable. This variability is abnormal when there are no indications that one of the variable pronunciations is potentially progressive, i.e. entails the possible development of a new contrast.

5   *Systematic sound preference* occurs when one type of consonant phone is used for a large range of different target types. Often, several different processes can be identified as resulting in a massive reduction of the phonological contrasts in the child's system: the processes 'conspire' to 'collapse' the adult system of contrasts to the one phone the child prefers to use in his or her pronunciation patterns: a 'favourite articulation'. The massive lack of contrasts is clearly indicative of a severe phonological learning disability, given the communicative inadequacies of the child's pronunciation patterns which must ensue (Grunwell, 1981, 1985b).

These characteristics identify the differences between normal and disordered development of phonology as displaying three types of developmental abnormality: delayed development; uneven development; deviant development. The occurrences of unequivocally deviant patterns in the speech of children with phonological disorders are usually only a minor aspect of the children's overall disordered pronunciation patterns. Furthermore, when these 'deviant' patterns are examined in detail, it is questionable whether or not they should be judged as such since it is often the case that equally unusual and essentially similar patterns occurring in much younger children, allegedly developing normally, are judged to be 'creative'. Thus it is primarily the chronological characteristics of delayed and uneven development that identify the developmental nature of phonological disorders.

These developmental characteristics also lead to insightful clinical evaluations of these disorders which provide the basis for an explanation of the nature of the children's learning difficulties. For example, Stoel-Gammon and Dunn (1985: 199) conclude that:

> phonological disorders could be characterized as a disorder involving the *process* of acquisition, thereby creating atypical patterns associated with the *product* of acquisition. According to this view, children with a phonological disorder proceed through the course of acquisition differently from normal children. In particular, children with phonological disorders seem to adhere to a different timetable for the emergence and mastery of sound and for the occurrence and suppression of phonological processes. For example, a disordered child may use a phonological process e.g. Final Consonant Deletion (which typically disappears early) at the same time that his inventory expands rapidly. As a result, the child would have a wide range of phones, but severely restricted range of syllable types, creating a system quite different from that of a normal child.

Leonard (1985: 8–9) provides an account which is complementary to Stoel-Gammon and Dunn's by hypothesizing in some detail as to how children with phonological disorders might arrive at unusual phonological behaviour in their pronunciation patterns. He takes as the starting point of his explanation the current cognitive model of children's phonological development:

> the child is viewed as an active learner who creates knowledge from the environmental input, rather than as a more passive learner whose acquisition of phonology is simply a linear progres-

sion of unfolding abilities. According to these models, the child stores for recognition some of the information available from the adult words spoken in the environment. This stored information does not necessarily preserve all the characteristics of the adult form. Differences between the child's stored form and the adult form may be the result of perceptual encoding rules or a failure to adequately store in memory less familiar though correctly perceived phonetic details. Output rules then relate the child's stored form for a word to his or her produced form. Importantly, these rules are both motivated and restricted by severe output constraints. These constraints may be the result of the child's limited ability to hit particular targets or to plan sequences of articulatory gestures. Of course, cases where accurately produced exceptions to a child's rule are subsequently produced less accurately to conform to the rule ... serve as examples that output rules can operate as organisational devices even in the absence of articulatory limitations. In any case, there are a number of ways in which an output constraint can be satisfied, and even children with limited articulatory control can devise solutions, albeit ones that may be limited in their range of application or in their communicative effectiveness.

It should be noted that Leonard's explanation requires the three-term model of speech production postulated by Hewlett (1985) and described above, in order to account for the different types of learning difficulties that children may experience in developing their phonological knowledge and pronunciation patterns.

Grunwell (1985c) also considers the developmental characteristics of these phonological disorders in the context of the current theoretical paradigm for child phonology and attempts a comprehensive explanation of the children's learning difficulties.

She suggests that as the children's pronunciation patterns are systematic and predictable they give evidence of rule formation. This view is reinforced by the fact that many of the patterns conform to those that children normally exhibit when beginning to learn to talk. Idiosyncratic or unusual patterns also occur. This, however, is further evidence of rule invention. It would appear from these characteristics that the children have problems in making progress in learning to pronounce. They seem to lack the ability to effect change in their pronunciation patterns and to devise new strategies to obtain and process information from the ambient language. The variability that is frequently observed in these children's speech provides further support to this interpretation. Variable pronunciation patterns suggest an inability to suppress several competing strategies and thus to effect systematic progressive changes in the organization of pronunciation.

Furthermore, it should be appreciated that these failures to make progress in phonological development have implications beyond the phonological level. The chronological mismatch is not limited to the internal phonological patterning. To a large extent the nature of the phonological disorder (i.e. the resultant unintelligible speech) is attributable to a mismatch between the potential of the child's phonology and the requirements of the other aspects of the child's productive language system. There is a mismatch between the communication needs of the child's syntax and semantics and the abilities of the phonological patterns to express those needs. The child's grammar and vocabulary have outgrown his or her phonology (Grunwell, 1981; see also Ingram, 1987). Thus the characteristic communicative inadequacy of the children's pronunciation patterns also has an essentially developmental explanation.

In this section we have considered the characteristics of children with developmental phonological disorders. We have described the phonetic and phonological tendencies identified in clinical populations of children with these disorders. It will be evident that these characteristics only enable us to identify the typical patterns in the data. In describing the developmental characteristics, however, we have also been able to put forward hypotheses as to why and how these phonomena have come about. These children may have processing and auditory–articulatory-analysis difficulties, or cognitive organizational restrictions, or problems in effecting reorganization of their phonetic motor-control programmes. Detailed investigation of each individual child will establish at which level/levels the breakdowns are occurring. We have discovered that their speech development has been in part normal and that their problems can be described in developmental terms. It is therefore in the context of a developmental description that we can begin to move towards an explanation of the nature of children's phonological learning difficulties. Furthermore, in conclusion, it should be noted that the developmental descriptive framework outlined here has also been used to assess and evaluate phonological disorders of children speaking languages other than English (specifically Brazilian Portuguese: Teixeira, 1986; Yavas, 1986; Swedish: Nettelbladt, 1983; Welsh: Munro, 1986), and similar characteristics have been identified.

CLINICAL ASSESSMENT PROCEDURES FOR DEVELOPMENTAL PHONOLOGICAL DISORDERS

The assessment procedures used for the clinical evaluation of developmental phonological disorders should be designed in such a way as to provide answers to the three questions outlined in the introductory section. More specifically they should fulfil the following clinical prerequisites:

1 The procedure should provide a description of the patterns in the child's pronunciation of spoken language; this description should be framed using both phonetic and phonological concepts and categories.

2 The procedure should identify the differences between the normal patterns of pronunciation and the patterns in the child's speech; that is, the phonetic and phonological differences between the adult and child speech.

3 The procedure should provide a framework in which to indicate the communicative implications of the child's patterns; this is the essentially phonological element of the assessment in that this framework evaluates the linguistic/functional consequences of the child's pronunciation patterns; i.e. the actual and implied failures to signal meaning differences through the lack of adequate phonological contrasts.

4 The procedure should provide a profile in which to evaluate the developmental status of the child's pronunciation patterns: this assessment provides the basis for a developmental diagnostic classification by identifying children who are different from normal children and distinguishing between children with delayed or uneven or deviant developmental profiles.

5 The procedure should facilitate the delineation of treatment aims and the planning of remediation programmes. In order to meet this requirement the procedure should contain frameworks and furnish guidelines for the prioritization of treatment targets. In addition, the theoretical framework underlying the descriptive assessment may inform the conceptualization of the remediation process.

6 Finally, the procedure should identify and evaluate changes in a child's pronunciation patterns when a second investigation is carried out for reassessment purposes; it is important to measure both the type and rate of change in children's speech in terms of communicative (functional) progress as well as developmental progress.

Currently the most popular approach to the assessment of children's phonological disorders is based on phonological process analysis. There are five widely known such procedures, all of which are specifically designed for the assessment of child speech. They are:

Weiner (1979), Phonological Process Analysis (PPA);
Shriberg and Kwiatkowski (1980), Natural Process Analysis (NPA);
Hodson (1980), Assessment of Phonological Processes (APP);
Ingram (1981), Procedures for the Phonological Analysis of Children's Language (PPACL);
Grunwell (1985b), Phonological Assessment of Child Speech (PACS).

In the latter two instances the phonological process analysis procedures are part of a set of procedures which involve a variety of different approaches to clinical phonological assessment. The other three procedures focus virtually exclusively on the process analysis as the main basis for the clinical assessment. Unfortunately, all five procedures employ ostensibly different sets of processes; these are listed in Table 2.1 (see pp. 52–3). On closer inspection, however, the similarity between the analytical frameworks becomes apparent; the differences being largely attributable to different classification systems and varying levels of detail in regard to the descriptive definitions of each process.

For example, in PPA, the processes are categorized into three types: *syllable-structure processes*; *harmony processes*; *feature-contrast processes*. This classification reflects that originally proposed by Ingram (1976) with minor changes in nomenclature; the original terms are syllable-structure processes; assimilatory processes; substitution processes. This classification is still in effect used by Ingram in PPACL, even though it is not specified:

Syllable-structure processes:
    deletion of final consonant;
    reduction of consonant clusters;
    syllable deletion and reduplication.
Substitution processes:
    fronting;
    stopping;
    simplification of liquids and nasals;
    other substitution processes.
Assimilation processes.

PACS employs a comparable, though significantly different, classificatory framework, categorizing processes according to whether they effect structural or systemic simplifications in children's speech by comparison with the adult pronunciation patterns. APP's classification shares some of the principles evident in the three procedures already considered, for example in distinguishing articulatory shifts (i.e. phonetic maturational pronunciation differences) from the other processes which involve phonemic differences and in identifying assimilations. The categorization into basic versus miscellaneous processes, however, appears to be somewhat *ad hoc*, especially when stopping is classified as a miscellaneous process.

Notwithstanding these classificatory and terminological differences, all five procedures operate with the same principles of analysis. Furthermore, the four procedures discussed so far consider the phonological processes in some detail and all are to a certain extent open-ended, in that they specifically allow for and encourage the analyst/clinician to identify other processes (see further below). In contrast, NPA is extremely limited in its range of processes, being restricted to eight, which, even though they are process categories rather than the detailed processes themselves, do not cover all the types of phonological simplifying relationships included in the other four procedures. 'Voicing' is in fact specifically excluded by the authors of NPA, as they claim it cannot be reliably transcribed and identified in child speech. In addition, no combinations of processes are allowed in the interpretation of the child's pronunciations; thus /kl/→[t] would be one process of cluster reduction, rather than the more transparent combination of cluster reduction and velar fronting. For these and other facets of the detailed applications of the NPA procedures, NPA is by far the least satisfactory of these five assessments (see further Grunwell 1987b).

All five procedures, nevertheless, share the same principles of description which lead to the same primary treatment aims. They all describe the systematic phonological relationships between adult and child pronunciation patterns, where they differ from each other, by reference to the selective aspects of the adult phonology identified by the theoretical framework of natural phonological processes. The clinical aim of all the assessments is primarily to lead to the implementation of a systematically structured therapy programme designed to facilitate progressive change in those aspects of a child's pronunciation where the processes are operative and which are therefore the target of therapy:

Table 2.1 Clinical assessment procedures using phonological-process analysis

Weiner (1979)	Shriberg and Kwiatkowski (1980)	Hodson (1980)
Syllable-structure process Deletion of final consonant cluster reductions: Initial stop + liquid Initial fricative + liquid Initial /s/ clusters Final /s/ + stop Final liquid + stop Final nasal + stop Weak-syllable deletion Glottal replacement	1 Final-consonant deletion 2 Velar fronting: Initial Final 3 Stopping: Initial Final 4 Palatal fronting: Initial Final	*Basic phonological processes* Syllable reduction Cluster reduction Prevocalic obstruent singleton omissions Postvocalic obstruent singleton omissions Stridency deletion Velar deviations
Harmony processes Labial assimilation Alveolar assimilation Velar assimilation Prevocalic voicing Final consonant devoicing	5 Liquid simplification: Initial Final 6 Assimilation: Progressive Regressive 7 Cluster reduction: Initial Final 8 Unstressed-syllable deletion	*Miscellaneous phonological processes* Prevocalic voicing Postvocalic devoicing Glottal replacement Backing Stopping Affrication Deaffrication Palatalization Depalatalization Coalescence Epenthesis Metathesis
Feature-contrast processes Stopping Gliding of fricatives Affrication Fronting Denasalization Gliding of liquids Vocalization		*Sonorant deviations* Liquid /l/ Liquid /rɚ/ Nasals Glides Vowels
		Assimilations Nasal Velar Labial Alveolar
		Articulatory Shifts Substitutions of /fvsz/ for /θð/ Frontal lisp Dentalization of /t d n l/ Lateralization

Ingram (1981)	*Grunwell (1985b)*	*Grunwell (1985b) cont.*

Deletion of final consonants
  1 Nasals
  2 Voiced stops
  3 Voiceless stops
  4 Voiced fricatives
  5 Voiceless fricatives
	Structural simplifications
	Weak-syllable deletion:
	  pretonic
	  posttonic
	Final consonant deletion:
	  nasals
	  plosives
	  fricatives
		Gliding:
		  /r/
		  /l/
		  fricatives

Reduction of consonant clusters
  6 Liquids
  7 Nasals
  8 /s/ clusters
	affricates
	  clusters − 1
	        − 2+
		Context-sensitive voicing:
		  WI and WF
		  Voicing WI
		  Voicing WW
		  Devoicing WF

Syllable deletion and reduplication
  9 Reduction of disyllables
 10 Unstressed-syllable deletion
 11 Reduplication
	Vocalization:
	  /l/
	  other C
	Reduplication:
	  complete
	  partial
	Consonant harmony:
	  velar
		Glottal replacement:
		  WI
		  WW
		  WF
		Glottal insertion

Fronting
 12 of palatals
 13 of velars
	alveolar
	  labial
	  manner
	  other	

Stopping
 14 of initial voiceless frics.
 15 of initial voiced frics.
 16 of initial affricates
	SI cluster reduction:
	  plosive+approximant
	  fricative+approximant
	  /s/+plosive
	  /s/+nasal
	  /s/+approximant
	  /s/+plosive+
	    approximant	

Simplification of liquids and nasals
 17 Liquid gliding
 18 Vocalization
 19 Denasalization
	Systemic simplifications
	Fronting:
	  velars
	  palato-alveolars	

Other substitution processes
 20 Deaffrication
 21 Deletion of initial consonants
 22 Apicalization
 23 Labialization
	Stopping:
	  /f/
	  /v/
	  /θ/
	  /ð/
	  /s/
	  /z/	

Assimilation processes
 24 Velar assimilation
 25 Labial assimilation
 26 Prevocalic voicing
 27 Devoicing of final consonants
	/ʃ/
	  /tʃ/
	  /dʒ/
	  /l/
	  /r/	

Simply stated, the phonological approach takes advantage of the systematic nature of speech deviations. Rather than focussing on individual sound errors and perfecting phoneme segments, the phonological approach attacks the basic system. Failure to produce /s/, for example, may be the result of different processes in different word situations ... remediating a phonological process in a young child's speech can influence all of the sounds that are similarly affected.... 'Acquiring new sound patterns' describes more accurately the way a child learns speech naturally rather than to say he is 'learning sounds'.

Phonology therefore provides a logical approach to training when the child has, for whatever reason, failed to acquire normal speech patterns on his own.

(Hodson and Paden, 1983: 5)

Although phonological process analysis has achieved its current position as the dominant approach to clinical assessment of child speech because of its use in studies of the normal development of phonology in children, there is only one of the five procedures that directly leads to a development assessment profile: PACS (see Figure 2.1). There is, however, quite detailed discussion of normal developmental patterns in both Shriberg and Kwiatkowski, and Ingram; but these discussions constitute descriptive accounts rather than normative profiles within which an individual child's pronunciation patterns could be measured and evaluated. With regard to the clinical evaluation of a child's pronunciation patterns, NPA, APP, PPACL and PACS all consider, in different ways, the characteristics of disordered use of phonological processes.

NPA includes an appendix in which clinical case studies of children with speech disorders are presented in some detail. APP covers in its list of processes unusual patterns such as glottal replacement, backing, nasal deviations. Ingram, in the manual for PPACL, describes and discusses the characteristics of disordered child phonology. Grunwell, in the PACS procedures and in the accompanying manual, provides the most comprehensive framework for a clinical evaluation of a phonological process assessment. In the PACS procedures themselves glottal realizations: replacement and insertions are specifically included to cater for these commonly occurring patterns in the speech of children with disordered development. In addition, there is provision for the detailed analysis of 'other' systemic and structural processes, which Grunwell indicates in the PACS manual (1985b: 58–9) are apparently unusual in the normally

Developmental Assessment

PACS
© Pamela Grunwell, 1985.
Published by
The NFER-NELSON Publishing Company Ltd.,
Darville House, 2 Oxford Road East, Windsor,
Berkshire SL4 1DF.

Name ....

		Labial	Lingual	Protowords and First Words:
Stage I (0;9 – 1;6)	Nasal			Show phonetic variability and all phon processes. *Examples*
	Plosive			
	Fricative			
	Approximant			

Stage II (1;6 – 2;0)					Reduplication, Consonant Harmony, FINAL CONS. DELETION, CLUSTER REDUCTION	FRONTING, STOPPING, GLIDING, C.S.VOICING
	m	n				
	p b	t d				
	w					

Stage III (2;0 – 2;6)					Final Cons. Deletion, CLUSTER REDUCTION	Fronting, STOPPING, GLIDING, C.S.VOICING
	m	n	(ŋ)			
	p b	t d	(k g)			
	w		(h)			

Stage IV (2;6 – 3;0)					Final Cons. Deletion, CLUSTER REDUCTION	STOPPING/v ð z tʃ dʒ/, FRONTING/ʃ/→[s], GLIDING, C.S.Voicing
	m	n	ŋ			
	p b	t d	k g			
	f	s				
	w	(l)	j	h		

Stage V (3;0 – 3;6)					Clusters used: obs. + approx. /s/ + cons.	STOPPING/v ð z/, FRONTING/ʃ tʃ dʒ/, GLIDING, /θ/→[f]
	m	n	ŋ			
	p b	t d (tʃ)	k g			
	f	s (ʃ)				
	w	l	j	h		

Stage VI (3;6 – 4;6)					Clusters used: obs. + approx. /s/ + cons.	/ð/→[d] or [v], PALATALIZATION/ʃ tʃ dʒ/, GLIDING, /θ/→[f]
	m	n	ŋ			
	p b	t d tʃ dʒ	k g			
	f v	s z ʃ				
	w	l (r)	j	h		

Stage VII (4;6 <)					Clusters used: obs. + approx. /s/ + cons.	/ð/→[d] or [v], /r/→[w] or [ʋ], /θ/→[f]
	m	n	ŋ			
	p b	t d tʃ dʒ	k g			
	f v θ	s ð z ʃ (ʒ)				
	w	l r	j	h		

Comments and Notes

_____

_____

_____

_____

_____

_____

_____

Figure 2.1

developing child population, or idiosyncratic to an individual child in either the normal or clinical context. Examples of the other processes illustrated include:

initial-consonant adjunction – the addition of a consonant before a word-initial vowel;

backing – the opposite of fronting; target alveolars pronounced as velars;

weakening (spirantization) of plosives to fricatives;

denasalization – target nasals pronounced as non-nasals.

PACS also provides a checklist of the characteristics of disordered child phonology, based on Grunwell (1981) and other researchers (e.g. Stoel-Gammon and Dunn, 1985). These characteristics are those described in the preceding section; viz. *persisting normal processes*; *chronological mismatch*; *unusual/idiosyncratic processes*; *variable use of processes*; *systematic sound preference.* There is not the space here to describe in detail each of the five procedures outlined in this section. Having established their shared similarities and significant differences in terms of the phonological process analysis, we shall now consider another important aspect for their construction: the elicitation procedures advocated by or required by the authors.

NPA, PPACL and PACS are all intended for use with spontaneous speech samples. NPA, however, is curiously restricted in this regard as the analytical procedure only fully analyses monosyllabic words, and only the first occurrence of those, thus excluding any possibility of detecting word-based variability in a child's pronunciation patterns. The other two procedures are designed to analyse all facets of a spontaneous speech sample, which for the purposes of phonological assessment should be: representative of the target phonology; representative of the habitual patterns used by the speaker; large enough to reveal variability (i.e. 200–50 words) homogeneous in time and type; glossed (see further Grunwell, 1985; PACS Pictures, 1987c).

Assessment of a spontaneous speech sample is much to be preferred and is therefore recommended in all possible circumstances. However, various factors, especially time constraints, may preclude this. Furthermore it is often necessary to structure the materials used to ensure that the sample elicited is representative (see PACS Pictures 1987c, for example). It is therefore understandable that the devisors of the other two procedures should choose *ab initio* to provide the samples for analysis. PPA and APP employ predeter-

mined elicitation procedures designed to obtain a specified sampl
one-word utterances. PPA is based on the presentation of pictures
elicit 136 words by cued naming and delayed imitation. APP uses a
set of twenty words in a screening version and fifty-five in the full
version, both sets being obtained largely through the meaning of a
collection of objects. It is also noteworthy that as well as the phonological process analysis procedure, PPA and NPA include an analysis
of the child's 'phonetic inventory', which is in effect a simple
checking-off procedure with regard to which English target consonant phonemes occur in the sample and whether or not they are
realized correctly.

As might be anticipated given the basic similarities of these procedures, assessments of children's speech are convergent when the
procedures are compared. This has been demonstrated for NPA,
APP and PPACL (Paden and Moss, 1985) and for selected processes
from APP and PPACL (Benjamin and Greenwood, 1983). For
further detailed discussion of these procedures see Grunwell (1987b).

While phonological process analysis undoubtedly occupies a
dominant position in the range of assessment procedures available to
the clinician at present, it should not be assumed that it is an entirely
satisfactory procedure. It can only identify those aspects of children's
pronunciation patterns that are different from the expected adult
pronunciations. Therefore, it is essentially a framework for identifying *error* patterns and does not as a consequence directly evaluate
the communicative implications of a child's mispronunciations. For
example, if a child's pronunciation errors involve the processes of
fronting of velars and stopping of fricatives and affricates, each of
these processes will be identified separately and there is no direct
mechanism within the procedure of making explicit that they entail
the following losses of contrasts:

$$/t/ \rightarrow [t]$$
$$/k/ \rightarrow [t]$$
$$/s/ \rightarrow [t]$$
$$/\int/ \rightarrow [t]$$
$$/\mathfrak{t}\int/ \rightarrow [t]$$

Once this limitation is acknowledged, then an informed and insightful
use of the procedures can result in identification of the implied
communicative inadequacies of the child's pronunciation patterns as
well as the phonological processes *per se* (see Leinonen-Davies,
1987).

Notwithstanding the possibilities for inventive use of process analysis in order to satisfy the prerequisites outlined above, it is preferable if an assessment procedure comprises a range of analytical techniques from which the clinician can select those which are most appropriate for the investigation of an individual child's pronunciation patterns. PACS (Phonological Assessment of Child Speech – Grunwell, 1985b) is such a procedure. As we have already seen PACS contains a phonological process analysis framework, but it also includes a wide variety of other procedures, the most important of which are:

The *phonetic inventory*: analysis of the phonetic range and distribution of consonant sounds occurring in the child's speech.
The *contrastive system* and the *phonotactic inventory*: analysis of the child's use of his or her phonetic inventory to signal meaning differences at different positions in word and syllable structure and the combinations of consonants that occur at these structural positions.

These two assessments, together with the process analysis, provide the information which enables the clinician to evaluate both the communicative adequacy and the developmental status of a child's pronunciation patterns. In PACS the main procedure for the evaluation communicative adequacy is the contrastive assessment (see Figure 2.2), which provides a direct comparison between the child and adult pronunciation systems. It should be noted that the contrastive analysis can also be matched against the PACS developmental assessment (see Figure 2.1) by entering the child's system of contrasts on the left-hand side of the profile. This capability reflects the flexibility of the PACS procedures.

There are a number of other assessment procedures that have appeared in the last decade specifically designed to analyse disordered child speech. It is the author's impression, however, that, despite highly prestigious origins, these procedures have not as yet been widely adopted in speech pathology practice or research in English-speaking communities. For this reason and because of space limitations they are not included in this in any event very brief review. Readers are referred directly to the procedures themselves (Ingram, 1981; Crystal, 1982; Elbert and Gierut, 1986) and to the summaries and reviews in Bernthal and Bankson (forthcoming), Edwards and Shriberg (1983) and Grunwell (1987b).

Systems of Contrastive Phones
and Contrastive Assessments

© Pamela Grunwell, 1985.
Published by
The NFER-NELSON Publishing Company Ltd.,
Darville House, 2 Oxford Road East, Windsor,
Berkshire SL4 1DF.

PACS

Name ....

Syllable Initial Word Initial

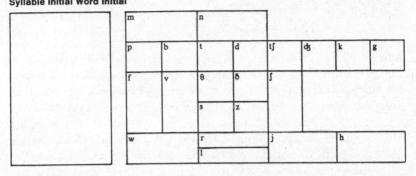

Syllable Initial Within Word

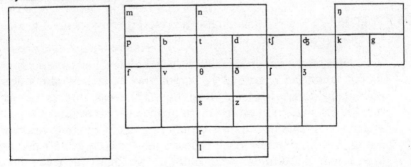

Syllable Final Word Final

Figure 2.2

FUNDAMENTAL CONCEPTS IN THE TREATMENT OF DEVELOPMENTAL PHONOLOGICAL DISORDERS

One of the primary aims of carrying out a phonological assessment of a child's speech patterns is to identify the targets of treatment. In our present state of knowledge, given the paucity of treatment studies, it is not possible to make definitive statements about how to select and order specific treatment goals or indeed to be confident of the very general guidelines that can be suggested. Be that as it may, the overriding goal of treatment can be readily stated: to facilitate an improvement in the child's ability to communicate through spoken language by promoting the necessary changes in his or her pronunciation patterns. This general aim focuses on the communicative rather than the developmental. This reflects the orientation of the author. Other authorities (for example, Hudson and Paden, 1983; Ingram, 1986) make the developmental framework the basis for the selection of treatment goals. Readers are referred to these texts for further information on the developmentally orientated approach to therapy. We shall be concentrating here on the communicative (or functional) approach.

As has been indicated in the outline of the characteristics of developmental phonological disorders, the children's pronunciation patterns are characterized by the following:

lack of contrasts required to signal meaning differences;
restrictions in combinations of phones, also required to signal meaning differences;
variability in pronunciations of target phonemes and individual words.

Of course, the pronunciation patterns that result in these characteristics will differ for each individual child. Nevertheless, general guidelines can be provided for each:

Variability entails unpredictability in pronunciation patterns and should therefore in general be 'eradicated'; but it is also often potentially progressive and when this is the case the variability should be stabilized to establish the incipient contrast.
The child's system of contrasts should be expanded; often this may not always involve introducing new sounds to the child's inventory; it may only require stabilization of variability (as mentioned above) or the extension of the use of an established phone to a new position in structure.
The child's range of possible consonant combinations should be

extended; this phonotactic dimension is often overlooked ⹁
therapy but it is very important to ensuring that the child's pronunciation patterns achieve greater communicative adequacy.

These three guidelines therefore summarize the prime targets for
phonological therapy. We shall finally consider premises and
principles of phonological therapy for children with developmental
phonological disorders. These are framed in the context of the
explanations of these disorders presented in the earlier sections of this
chapter. It is assumed that the objective is to assist the child to acquire
the adult pronunciation system by focusing on the organization and
communicative functions of that system. It is also assumed that this
approach is necessary because the child has been unable to learn that
system alone given normal exposure to the ambient language. Therefore, a structured presentation of those dimensions of the system that
he or she has failed to learn is required. Thus the treatment procedures themselves, which will not be discussed here (see further
Grunwell, 1985b, 1987b), will focus on a particular function dimension of the adult pronunciation system and will also manipulate the
child's linguistic environment to ensure a more concentrated exposure to this dimension.

As Grunwell (1983) established, the fundamental premise of
phonological therapy is that the changes to be facilitated in the child's
pronunciation patterns are primarily changes in the child's knowledge
of the phonology of his or her language. The aim of treatment is to
effect cognitive reorganization rather than articulatory retraining.
Therapy strategies should therefore focus on exposing the child's
communicative inadequacies in a systematic way as a means to
improve his or her communicative abilities.

Premises of phonological therapy

These are the theoretical bases from which phonological therapy has
developed. They reflect assumptions about the nature of phonology
and of children's phonological development summarized in the earlier
section of this chapter.

1   The child has a phonological learning disorder – therapy must be
     aimed at remediating this cognitive and organizational disorder,
     not at training motor skills for the articulation of speech sounds;
     though for some children this may be necessary too.
2   In learning his or her phonological system, a child is developing a
     system of sound contrasts which signal meaning differences –

therapy must therefore use spoken language, i.e.
medium of communication.

his phonology, a child is organizing his phonological
. he is not just learning the correct pronunciation of
words; he is discerning similarities between contrastive sounds
and sound sequences, which provide the bases for grouping
sounds into classes and sequences into structures. Activities in
therapy should promote this type of learning.

4   The aim of therapy is therefore to facilitate cognitive reorganization of the child's phonological system and his phonologically
orientated processing strategies – as every child has a different
system when he or she enters therapy and is assumed to operate
with to a certain extent idiosyncratic processing strategies, each
remediation programme must be individually planned to address
the phonological difficulties of each child.

Principles of phonological therapy

These are statements of the operational policy of the therapeutic
approach and provide the explicit motivation for the selection of
specific treatment procedures. These principles are derived from the
premises listed above.

1   The treatment programme is based on a phonological analysis
and assessment. Goals of treatment are defined by this analysis
and assessment.
2   Therapy is based on the principle that there are patterns or regu-
larities in the child's spoken language.
3   Therapy is based on the principle that the principal function of
phonological patterning is communicative; i.e. to signal meaning
differences.
4   Therapy aims to change the child's phonological patterns in order
to build up a more adequate system of sound contrasts and sound
structures.
5   Therapy is designed to make maximally effective use of the
organization of phonological patterning by introducing and
establishing changes in the child's patterns through employing
natural classes of contrastive phones and structures. (based on
Grunwell, 1985b).

These premises and principles establish unequivocally the need for a
phonological analysis and assessment as the basis for the treatment of
phonological disorders in children. They also indicate the necessity

for further studies of the nature of phonological development both normal and disordered, so that we can achieve a better understanding of the learning mechanism and processes involved when children are learning or sadly failing to learn to pronounce.

REFERENCES

Benjamin, B.J. and Greenwood, J. (1983) 'A comparison of three phonological assessment procedures', *Journal of Childhood Communication Disorders*, vol. VII: 19–27.

Bernthal, J.E. and Bankson, N.W. (1987) *Articulation Disorders* 1st edn 1981; 2nd edn forthcoming, Englewood Cliffs, NJ: Prentice Hall.

Crystal, D. (1982) *Profiling Linguistic Disability*, London: Edward Arnold.

Edwards, M.L. and Shriberg, L.D. (1983) *Phonology: Applications in Communicative Disorders*, San Diego: College Hill.

Elbert, M. and Gierut, J. (1986) *Handbook of Clinical Phonology*, London: Taylor and Francis.

Grunwell, P. (1981) *The Nature of Phonological Disability in Children*, London: Academic Press.

Grunwell, P. (1983) 'Phonological therapy: premises, principles and procedures', in *Proceedings of International Association of Logopaedics and Phoniatrics Congress*, Edinburgh.

Grunwell, P. (1985a) 'Comment on the terms "phonetics" and "phonology" as applied in the investigation of speech disorders', *British Journal of Disorders of Communication* 20: 165–70.

Grunwell, P. (1985b) *Phonological Assessment of Child Speech (PACS)* Windsor: NFER-Nelson.

Grunwell, P. (1985c) 'Developing phonological skills', *Child Language Teaching and Therapy* 1: 65–72.

Grunwell, P. (1986) 'Aspects of phonological development in later childhood', in K. Durkin (ed.) *Language Development During the School Years*, London: Croom Helm, 34–56.

Grunwell, P. (1987a) 'Evaluation and explanation of developmental phonological disorders', paper presented at the first AFASIC International Symposium on Specific Speech and Language Disorders in Children, University of Reading, UK.

Grunwell, P. (1987b) *Clinical Phonology*, 2nd edn, London: Croom Helm.

Grunwell, P. (1987c) *PACS Pictures*, Windsor: NFER-Nelson.

Grunwell, P. (1987d) 'Phonological assessment and evaluation of child speech', paper given at Communicative Workshop, Fourth International Congress for the Study of Child Language, University of Lund, Sweden.

Grunwell, P. and Russell, J. (1987) 'Phonological development in cleft palate children', paper given at Fourth International Congress for the Study of Child Language, University of Lund, Sweden.

Hewlett, N. (1985) 'Phonological versus phonetic disorders: some suggested modifications to the current use of the distinction', *British Journal of Disorders of Communication* 20: 155–64.

Hodson, B.W. (1980) *The Assessment of Phonological Processes*, Danville, Il: Interstate.

Hodson, B.W. and Paden, E.P. (1983) *Targetting Intelligible Speech*, San Diego: College Hill.

Ingram, D. (1976) *Phonological Disability in Children*, London: Edward Arnold.

Ingram, D. (1981) *Procedures for the Phonological Analysis of Children's Language*, Baltimore: University Park Press.

Ingram, D. (1986) 'Explanation and phonological remediation', *Child Language Teaching and Therapy* 2: 1–16.

Ingram, D. (1987) 'Categories of phonological disorder', plenary paper given at the first AFASIC International Symposium on Specific Speech and Language Disorders in Children, University of Reading, UK.

Leinonen, E. (1987) 'Assessing the functional adequacy of children's phonological systems', CNAA PhD thesis, Leicester Polytechnic.

Leonard, L.B. (1985) 'Unusual and subtle phonological behavior in the speech of phonological disordered children, *Journal of Speech and Hearing Disorders* 50: 4–13.

Munro, S. (1986) 'Phonological and morphological disorders in bilingual Welsh- and English-speaking children', PhD thesis, University of Wales.

Nettelbladt, U. (1983) *Developmental Studies of Dysphonology in Children*, Lund: CWK Gleerup.

Paden, E.P. and Moss, S.A. (1985) 'Comparison of three phonological analysis procedures', *Language Speech and Hearing Services in Schools* 16: 103–9.

Schwartz, R.G., Leonard, L.B., Wilcox, M.J. and Folger, M.K. (1980) 'Early phonological behavior in normal-speaking and language-disordered children: evidence for a synergistic view of language disorders', *Journal of Speech and Hearing Disorders* 45: 357–77.

Shriberg, L.D. and Kwiatkowski, J. (1980) *Natural Process Analysis (NPA)*, New York: John Wiley.

Stoel-Gammon, C. and Dunn, C. (1985) *Normal and Disordered Phonology in Children*, Baltimore, MD: University Park Press.

Teixeira, E.R. (1986) 'Developmental phonological disorders in Brazilian Portuguese', PhD thesis, University of London.

Yavas, M. (1986) 'Phonological developmental disorders in children learning Brazilian Portuguese', unpublished paper.

Weiner, F.F. (1979) *Phonological Process Analysis (PPA)*, Baltimore, MD: University Park Press.

3 Interactions among language components in phonological development and disorders

Richard G. Schwartz

Our natural tendencies to label, to categorize and to compartmentalize frequently lead us astray in dealing with systems that are not genuinely independent. This is often true of phonology and other components of language. In description, assessment and intervention there is typically a marked division among language components. Certainly, some of this reflects a natural and appropriate focus of attention. However, in many cases, understanding the interactions of language components is critical to our understanding of disordered speech and, more practically, to assessment and intervention.

Despite increased use of samples of spontaneous, connected speech for phonological analyses, speech-language pathologists and developmental phonologists have not taken advantage of the potential for examining other aspects of language along with phonology. Typically, even the most obvious opportunity is lost. Despite the longer, more complex, utterances in such samples, the standard approach to phonological analysis involves separating these utterances into single words. Thus, any information about a syntax–phonology interaction is lost.

The nature of these language interactions is potentially quite complex. For example, if we consider only pairwise possibilities, three language components (e.g., syntax, semantics, phonology) yields six possibilities with direction of influence taken into account. If we divide language into a greater number of components or add the possibility of three-way interactions, the number of possibilities increases rapidly (see Crystal, 1987, for a discussion). Adding to the potential complexity are the consideration of both input (comprehension and perception) and production abilities as well as individual differences. Finally, there are, as Crystal noted, interactions between phonology and phonetics as well as between segmental and suprasegmental units. To make all this manageable I will focus on those interactions that have been documented or seem most likely to be encountered in clinical populations. However, I hope to point also to some new possibilities derived from descriptions of normal development, psycholinguistic experiments and theoretical proposals.

An appropriate starting point is to consider the role of such interactions in linguistic and psycholinguistic theory. Despite continued support for the autonomy of language components in theoretical and in processing models, a shift in acceptance of interactive characterizations seems to have occurred. Some recent advances in phonological theory have pointed to phonological–syntactic relationships, suprasegmental–segmental interaction. The most recent versions of phonological theory (see Hogg and McCully, 1987, for a review) present a much more detailed description of the interaction between phonology and syntax than was offered by the box and line drawings of earlier generative phonology. The major points of departure are the treatment of stress and the attention given to the syllable. In generative phonology stress was dealt with at the level of the segment. Newer phonological theories emphasize the syllables as the primary unit and some also include units such as phonological words (which do not necessarily correspond to orthographic/semantic words) and phrases. A primary focus of these theories is the assignment of stress or prominence. The elements of structure are a grid which represents hierarchical patterns of syllable prominence and a tree structure which, following certain constraints, assigns strong and weak syllables to output in a branching fashion. All of this is tied intimately to syntactic structure. In one particular proposal (Selkirk, 1984), there are 'Text-to-Grid Alignment' rules that map word and phrase stress from surface syntax to phonological rules. Thus, the tie between syntax and phonology, though still unidirectional is much more explicit than in generative phonology.

Though I will present descriptive data from a single child (Stemberger, 1988) whose errors could be characterized in a syllable framework, much of this theoretical work is still somewhat promissory for child phonology and certainly for clinical applications. However, for those children whose errors do not neatly fit into a traditional word-based or exclusively segmental phonology, such advances will be very important.

Another source of theoretical advances is recent psycholinguistics work in the areas of sentence production and spoken-word recognition. In sentence production, the models have shifted from black box and arrow models to more detailed descriptions of the processes involved (e.g. Bock, 1982, 1987; Dell, 1986). Furthermore, the relationships among components of language are viewed as potentially bidirectional and determined by linguistic, cognitive and motoric factors. This yields a richer, but substantially more complex picture of sentence production. It has also yielded newer methodologies and emphasized data sources such as speech errors as a means of examining these processes. We have yet to see these methods and data sources applied to normally developing or disordered children. However, when they are applied they may clarify some of the relationships addressed in this chapter.

The other relevant area in which there have been substantial advances is that of speech perception/word recognition. This area has seen the merger of two lines of research: speech perception and spoken-word recognition. In speech perception the emphasis has been on the processing of acoustic stimuli as well as the discrimination, identification and perception of phonetic and phonemic stimuli. A majority of experiments in this line of research have employed stimuli that are not meaningful (e.g. syllables). A parallel line of research has considered the processing of acoustic and phonetic information but has focused on the recognition of spoken words and in some cases larger units (e.g. Grosjean and Gee, 1987; Marslen-Wilson, 1987). In these models factors such as the word prominence or stress in a phrase, phonological structure and phonetic content play a key role in word recognition and linguistic processing. As in the case of the sentence-production models, these models also incorporate structures such as spreading activation, strength of activation and bidirectional influences among linguistic levels. Speech perception is directed to a large degree by the top-down information of contextual syntax and semantics. Lexical recognition may be driven bottom-up by phonetic and phonological information as well as by syntactic information.

From a common-sense standpoint, one might expect relationships among language components simply because children do not learn aspects of language in isolation. One important issue to consider is that historically, the relationship has been viewed as a top-down relationship with phonology at the bottom. As the evidence indicates, though, this may not always be the case. We will consider the relationship between syntax and phonology and between the lexicon and phonology.

Evidence of interactions between phonology and other aspects of language are extensive. For the sake of organization, we can divide this large body of evidence into three areas: (1) the co-ordination of development and of disorders across the components of language; (2)

the on-line relationship across components of language; and (3) relationships within phonology between segmental and suprasegmental factors and between phonetics and phonology. The chapter will focus on the first two areas; coverage of the third will be incidental, with some attention in the course of discussing other areas (e.g. phonology and information level). The chapter will also be unbalanced in its emphasis on syntax and phonology. This simply reflects the relative investigation attention to this interaction as compared to other relationships.

INTERACTIONS IN DEVELOPMENT AND DISORDERS

The co-ordination of development and disorders across language components has long been known. However, the specifics of these relationships can be varied and puzzling. Understanding the co-occurrence of disorders across language components may prove very valuable in making an accurate assessment and in providing some differential approaches to intervention. We have long had evidence that children identified as language-impaired have deficits in speech production as well as perception and conversely that children identified as having speech-sound disorders have difficulty with other aspects of language, notably syntax (see Crystal, 1988, for a review). These studies have taken several forms. In one approach children identified as articulation-disordered or language-impaired are given some type of task to assess their abilities in another domain of language and perform poorly. Unfortunately, this is not particularly informative. Another type of investigation is one in which normal and disordered children are matched on some measure of language (usually MLU) and their production abilities are compared along some other dimension. Such investigations have been common in other areas. They have less commonly involved phonology. One such investigation examined the phonologies of three normally developing children and three language-impaired children who were matched for MLU and cognitive abilities (Schwartz *et al.*, 1980). Across a number of independent and relational measures we found that these children had very similar phonetic inventories (sounds and word structures of the child's productions), selection characteristics (sounds and word structures in the adult targets), error patterns, inter- and intraword variability. Despite the small number of subjects, it is clear that at this early point in development (these children were all at a single-word utterance level), holding MLU constant yielded equivalent phonologies, regardless of the children's differences in chronological age.

This indicated, rather convincingly, that early in development advances disorders in phonology and syntax were tied together.

A subsequent examination of speech-disordered children revealed a great deal more detail about the co-occurrence of phonological, morphological and syntactic deficits (Paul and Shriberg, 1982). Several patterns of association were used to describe the children's speech (see Table 3.1). Approximately two-thirds of these speech-delayed children exhibited syntactic deficits (Patterns I and III) that are not just omission of grammatical morphemes because of unstressed-syllable deletion or final-consonant deletion. Twenty per cent of the children exhibited morphological delays that were the result of phonological disabilities involving the aforementioned errors. The remaining children (Pattern IV) did not exhibit any syntactic or morphological delay. As we might expect, speech-disordered children are not a homogeneous group and concomitant or causally related disorders in other aspects of language vary in their occurrence. Teasing out these relationships is important in understanding the nature of phonological disorders and in approaching intervention for these children. Clearly the nature of intervention will differ markedly for the children with different profiles.

The co-occurrence of deficits has not received as much attention as is needed to understand the full range of possibilities. If we are to assess and intervene with speech-language disordered children in an integrated fashion then we need more information. An important

Table 3.1 Patterns of association between phonology and syntax

Pattern I	The child has an overall syntactic delay and a greater delay in the production of morphemes that are phonetically complex (i.e., plural, possessive, regular past tense and regular third-person singular, because in English these increase the surface complexity of the rules).
Pattern II	The child exhibits a level of syntactic production that is age-appropriate, but deficits in the production of complex morphophonemes.
Pattern III	The child has a general syntactic deficit, but grammatical morphemes are produced adequately, relative to the child's level of syntactic development.
Pattern IV	The child's abilities in both areas are within normal limits.

Source: Adapted from Paul and Shriberg (1982).

source is the on-line processing interactions and the influence of these interactions on immediate behaviour as well as on the course of development. I will explore these relationships in the next section. Because the information from speech-language-impaired (SLI) children is limited, we will extrapolate where possible in discussing the implications of these interactions for clinical activities.

ON-LINE PROCESSING

One phenomenon observed in both normal and SLI children is that increases in complexity in one domain seem to have a cascading effect on other domains of language behaviour. Other related observations concern the nature of speech errors in children and the course of development that may result from on-line processing considerations. Most, though not all, of these data come from normally developing children. I will divide the data, somewhat arbitrarily, by language component and conclude by a discussion of the implications for SLI children.

Lexical selection

One of the more obvious relationships between phonology and other components of language involves a phenomenon of early development termed 'selectivity'. The gaps observed in young children's production lexicons can be characterized as following phonological patterns (Ferguson and Farwell, 1975; Schwartz and Leonard, 1982). It appears that children predominantly choose to produce words with targets that are consistent with sounds they produce correctly most of the time. There are some patterns consistent across children; however, there are also some substantive individual differences.

Over the last ten years (see Schwartz, 1988, for a review), Laurence Leonard and I (along with a number of colleagues) have studied lexical selectivity in both normal and language-impaired children using an experimental procedure in which we obtain a sample of the child's speech and identify two types of consonants – IN and OUT (Leonard *et al.*, 1982; Schwartz and Leonard, 1982). IN consonants are those which the child produces correctly in a majority of cases (about 67 per cent) and OUT consonants are those that did not occur either in adult targets or in the child's production (either as correct productions or as substitutions for other sounds). These sounds were then used to choose a set of unfamiliar words or to construct a set of unfamiliar words. The IN and OUT words were then presented along with their referents an equal number of times in utterance-final position (e.g., 'Here's the *bok*') during about ten sessions over a period of about three to four weeks. These selectivity characteristics did not seem to influence children's comprehension; IN and OUT words are comprehended in equal numbers. The status of a word did, however, make a significant difference in the children's likelihood of production. IN words were produced in significantly greater numbers than OUT words by normally developing children with production vocabularies of as few as three words to children with vocabularies as high as seventy-five words. We have also found that experimental words constructed on the basis of babbling characteristics (i.e., IN sounds) are acquired in greater numbers than experimental words consisting of sounds that were not produced (Messick, 1984). It is quite apparent that during the period of the first 50–100 words children's lexical acquisition is, at least in part, driven by phonological factors. Children who have clear selection strategies and a small set of preferred articulatory routines may exhibit more rapid lexical acquisition than children who are more diffuse in their selection characteristics and more varied in their output patterns (Stoel-Gammon and Cooper, 1984).

We have recently extended the paradigm to include a third category of words, ATTEMPTED (Leonard *et al.*, 1987; Schwartz *et al.*, 1987). These words include consonants that have occurred as targets in the child's productions, but have not been produced correctly according to parent report and our initial sample. Consistent with our previous findings, there were no comprehension effects. ATTEMPTED words were similar to OUT words in the likelihood with which they were produced. When normally developing children produced these words, they tended to make the same errors that we had observed in their initial samples. However, when SLI children produced these words, the errors seemed to be independent of their existing production patterns. Thus disordered children do seem to be more limited in behaving within a phonologically organized lexicon.

There is even some evidence that the influence of selectivity extends to early syntactic development. Donahue (1986) reported that her son had already just begun producing two-word utterances (e.g. *no ball*, *no dog*, *bye bird*, *bye daddy*), when a pattern of consonant harmony (for place of articulation) and strong selection preference for bilabials first appeared in single lexical items. The two-word utterances were short-lived. When they reappeared three months later, several characteristics were apparent: first, his two-word utterances were consistent with the selection preferences and consonant-harmony rule evidenced in the single-word productions; he also added pivot words that were produced vocalically (so they did not conflict with his consonant-harmony constraint); finally, as velar harmony became more frequent in single-word productions it spread to two-word utterances. Two-word utterances that were outside this child's selection preferences or could not be operated on by the consonant-harmony rule were simply not produced, despite some frequent parental prompting.

Thus selectivity seems to play a significant role in directing the nature and rate of early lexical acquisition and perhaps early word combinations. To be sure, phonology interacts with facts such as semantics, communicative needs and rudimentary syntax in forming the course of early development. Although motor development may account for some changes in selection and production, other factors are likely to play a significant role in pressing the child gradually to violate any narrow selection patterns that might exist. It is apparent that selection must be taken into account in any planning for assessment or intervention aimed at children in this developmental period.

Lexical type

A second aspect of lexical use and acquisition concerns lexical type. Children consistently exhibit a bias in favour of object words early in language. They are acquired in greater numbers and earlier than most other word types. Normal and language-impaired children produce [s] more accurately in object words than in action words (Cohen, 1978). At first glance, this type of difference might be difficult to explain. However, a number of differences between these two word types might account for this type of finding. Object words may be more salient in input because they tend to occur at the end or beginning of utterances or as single-word utterances, whereas verbs tend to be embedded in the sentence. Object words may be more frequent in input. Also, the fact that verbs can take a greater variety of morphological affixes than nouns may make their stems harder to segment and identify. In order to control for some of these factors Camarata and Schwartz (1985) followed an examination of normal and language-impaired children's speech (single-word utterance users) with an experimental nonsense-word experiment. In both cases the children produced the object words more accurately than the action words. In a follow-up study of normal children, the findings were confirmed with a larger number of words (Camarata and

Leonard, 1986). The children's productions of action words involved developmentally earlier errors, and new consonants were attempted only in object words.

The explanation for the differences cannot lie in any asymmetry or advantage for object words in input because of the control offered by the nonsense-word procedure. Instead, some inherent differences between object and action words must be responsible for these findings. Object words are conceptually and perceptually simpler than action words in the nature of their referents. Object referents are perceptually stable and represent, at most, a class of objects. In contrast, verb referents may not be concrete or stable (often what is left perceptually is the result of the action or state change, not the referent) and represent a relationship, minimally between an actor and some movement or state change. Furthermore, in some cases, an object referent may be conceptually simpler in that it is included in a verb referent (e.g., *roll* refers to the object referent of *ball* moving in a particular way). Given this difference Camarata and his co-workers argued that at this early point in development this increase in conceptual complexity apparently has a significant impact on the child's limited-capacity system leading to a greater number of production errors.

This raises some serious clinical concerns regarding assessment and intervention for children at this level. The bias in tests and therapy materials favouring nouns may adversely affect the representativeness of assessment samples and the generalization of intervention results.

Syntax

Investigators (e.g. de Villiers and de Villiers, 1978) have observed in one child words that were produced accurately as single-word utterances but contained errors when they were included in multiword productions. Waterson (1978) reported that as her son produced longer utterances during the course of development he reverted to more familiar, established sounds and a lower degree of phonological differentiation (a complex measure taking into account the number of words, syllables, phonological contrasts and new articulations). It is also common to hear reports from parents who describe decreases in intelligibility of their children's speech that are concomitant with spurts in syntactic development. An additional point to consider is the suggestion (Branigan, 1979) that the transition between successive single-word utterances and true two-word utterances, sometimes termed successive single-word utterances, is dependent on motor-speech factors (i.e., the ability to produce a single, co-ordinated rhythm or intonation contour).

Phonologically disordered children exhibit the same phenomenon: often, children who can produce sounds quite accurately in isolated words become unintelligible in connected speech (see e.g., Faircloth and Faircloth, 1970).

Though these observations are intriguing, they fall short of demonstrating a direct syntax–phonology link. Some more systematic evidence has been offered by Panagos and his colleagues (see Panagos, 1982, for a review; Prelock, 1982). The paradigm has typically involved asking children to imitate a series of linguistic stimuli varying in syntactic complexity (e.g. isolated noun phrases, as well as active, passive and embedded sentences) and phonological complexity (typically defined in terms of the number of syllables). Across these experiments, increases in syntactic complexity led to syntactic errors (e.g. word omissions) and to phonological errors (e.g. substitutions or omissions). Increases in phonological complexity also resulted in both syntactic and phonological errors. These results have to be interpreted cautiously because of a number of limitations in the stimuli and in the paradigm. Among some of the problems are the following: (1) some of the sentences were quite complex, perhaps beyond the children's comprehension abilities and thus not representative of normal sentence production; (2) there was a confound between sentence length and syntactic complexity and a likely confound between word length and familiarity; (3) errors, particularly in the production of speech sounds, were not evaluated to determine whether they actually represented structural or developmental simplifications.

More recently, another set of experiments have added to this body of literature by examining younger children and in some cases comparing spontaneous productions with imitative productions (Kamhi *et al.*, 1984; Nelson and Kamhi, 1984; Masterson and Kamhi, 1985). These investigations addressed some, but not all of the above-mentioned limitations. In the first, children approximately two years of age were seen for a series of sentence-imitation sessions over a period of four months. The sentences included a single word, modifier + noun, subject–verb–object (SVO), SVO + subject modifier, SVO + negative contraction, yes–no questions with *did* and two passives. The children varied in their use of these sentence types. Phonological complexity was manipulated by using target words with late-emerging sounds (e.g. /ʒ ʃ dʒ/) as well monosyllabic and disyllabic words (e.g. *jar, sausage*). Analyses based on the consistency of target-word production were added by Panagos and his colleagues to the overall percentage of consonants correctly used. In contrast to previous studies, the results were very mixed, indicating differential effects of complexity increases across developmental stages and within stages across children. Increases in linguistic complexity had no effect in most cases. In cases where there was an effect, accuracy was as likely to increase as it was to decrease. Closer examination of the findings did reveal some influence of complexity increases on accuracy for the less advanced children, perhaps the result of the greater variability seen in the productions of these children. An even greater difference than this developmental discrepancy emerged from comparisons of children at the same level of linguistic development. Within a level of language development, some children exhibited greater variability than other children. This extended across stimulus conditions so that there was an association of increased linguistic complexity on children who are more tolerant of variability.

Interestingly, in a follow-up study using nonsense words as targets, Nelson and Kamhi (1984) did find that as syntactic complexity increased, phonetic accuracy in imitations decreased. Furthermore, these effects were also seen in spontaneous speech, but only during transitional periods of syntactic growth. A somewhat broader-scope study with older children (Masterson and Kamhi, 1985) also provided evidence of some specific interactions. Sentences containing complex phonological forms were shorter and contained more phonetic and grammatical errors than sentences containing simple phonological forms. The number of words judged to be unintelligible in limited sentences increased with phonological complexity increases in complex or embedded sentences. When the sentences were right- or centre-embedded and contained phonologically complex words, there were a great number of disfluencies. In general, the normally developing children exhibited fewer errors than either the language-impaired or reading-disabled children included in this study. One of the more notable differences between the language-impaired and the reading-disabled students was the poorer phonetic accuracy of the language-impaired children.

The inconsistencies across studies may be attributed to several factors. The small number of subjects employed, coupled with the substantial individual differences may explain this variation. I am also not convinced that we have yet to establish the best approach to measuring these effects. Some may be quite subtle and will require ingenious methodologies to yield the effects of interest and yet not artificial behaviours unrelated to normal sentence production. For now, however, it seems safe to conclude that phonology and syntax are related in sentence production under certain circumstances.

Some recent confirmation of this relationship comes from a study of adult sentence production that examined the influence of phonological priming on sentence production. Bock (1987) found that by having subjects silently read or say aloud a word similar to a target word in its initial sound and rhyme it had some inhibiting effect on target-word production. Specifically, in constructing a sentence following this priming, the primed word tended to be placed later in the produced sentence than the unprimed word. The fact that these effects occur following silent reading of the word suggests that it may represent a higher-level phonological effect.

There are at least two plausible explanations for these phenomena. One is simply the impact of motor overloading by adding more syllables to the target production. Although this has not been ruled out as a factor, it is unlikely to account for all of the findings to date. A second explanation relies on the limited-capacity model proposed by Panagos and his colleagues and some related models. According to this proposal, during sentence production there is an interaction between syntactic and phonological processes such that increases in complexity to either component disrupts the other and the cumulative complexity leads to performance disruption in both domains. The end result is typically simplification. The main idea is an interesting one. Despite the specification of a hierarchical relationship, it is not empirically distinguishable from Crystal's 'bucket' proposal. In this metaphor, if the bucket is filled beyond capacity, it will overflow (sometimes a drop at a time) and the result may be something with which the speaker and, perhaps, the listener must deal. It is also generally consistent with a, now old, version of Bock's (1982) model of sentence production. In this model she includes several relevant notions, among them the importance of factors such as processing capacity and automaticity. Automaticity is particularly important because more automatic behaviours require fewer processing resources. It is a notion that fits well with many of these data. If children have some difficulty with more complex, less familiar words, with more complex syntactic structures, with new syntactic structures during periods of rapid developmental advances or even with longer utterances (when more typical utterances are shorter) it may be in some way attributable to automaticity. In more recent versions some models rely on parallel processing (e.g. Dell, 1986; Bock, 1987) and spreading-activation types of architecture. This replaces a unidirectional top-down model with one that allows feedback from lower levels to upper levels of a sentence-production system. Consequently, these models are better able to explain the bidirectional influence of linguistic factors. Activation levels may be used to account for the relative automaticity of certain output units.

As the specificity and accuracy sentence-production models improve, we may also gain insight into the nature of the disruptions of the system, particularly those in speech- and language-impaired children. For now, an awareness of the nature of these interactions should direct our assessment towards their discovery in individual children, particularly as a potential source of variability and our intervention programming to take advantage of facilitating effects and to avoid complexity effects.

Between-word errors and connected-speech characteristics

Despite the use of connected-speech samples to analyse children's error patterns, all of our current procedures examine words one by one to determine the error patterns present. Thus, despite the fact that such samples allow for the effects of producing sounds in connected speech, none of the errors identified ever are associated with any factors outside the word. Some of the more recent phonological theories mentioned earlier as well as several other syllable-orientated proposals provide a framework within which we can consider processes that go beyond the boundaries of a single lexical item. In a diary study of his daughter, Stemberger (1988) described eight such patterns. The eight were:

1   word-final resyllabification – the final sound in one word becomes the initial sound in the following word when the second word begins with a vowel;
2   *h*-fusion – a resyllabification that also affected words beginning with *h*;
3   /l/-doubling – an /l/ or a substitution for it is carried over and doubled from the end of one syllable to the beginning of the next either within a word or across word boundaries;
4   vowel deletion – when two vowels come together at a word boundary one is deleted;
5   word-final nasal assimilation – the nasal at the end of one word assimilates to the beginning of the next word;
6   word-initial deletion of the voiced *th* (/ð/) – occurred only following words that ended in /n/ and involved specific words;

7   closed-class reduplication – the child's replacement of the utter-
ance-initial unstressed closed-class lexical item with reduplicated
consonants from the following word;

8   labiodental harmony – perseverative or anticipatory change of a
bilabial to a labiodental consonant.

Stemberger's observations represent a first step. It remains to be seen
how common such patterns are in other normally developing children
as well as in disordered populations. I suspect we will find them to be
fairly common oncé we begin to look beyond word boundaries. For
example, a child we recently saw in our clinic exhibited a pattern of
velar perseverative harmony in connected speech. Discovering these
patterns will provide a better description of children's phonologies,
more appropriate intervention procedures, and may help to explain
why a given word might be produced one way in a particular context
and differently in another context.

Syntactic conditioning of phonetic form comes from two additional
areas: suprasegmental characteristics and certain types of speech
errors. Adults lengthen words at the end of phrases (Klatt, 1975;
Sorenson *et al.*, 1978) and exhibit a greater drop in fundamental
frequency before strong (major) syntactic boundaries than weak ones
(Cooper and Sorenson, 1981).

It is not uncommon to hear reports of the speech of disordered
children who seem to have atypical connected speech. Such observations may be the result of variation in stress and prosody. Among
some of the findings include changes in fundamental frequency at
pause boundaries and phrase- or sentence-final lengthening. These
features have not yet been examined in either disordered or normally
developing populations. Given findings concerning the effect of stress
(reflecting changes in fundamental frequency, duration and intensity)
on accuracy (see below), there may be some complex interactions
among segmental accuracy, syntactic characteristics and supra-
segmentals.

Sound-exchange errors or spoonerisms (e.g. *Fats and Kodor* for
Katz and Fodor; see Fromkin, 1973) reveal another aspect of the
relationship between phonology and syntax in on-line processing.
Such errors are influenced by similarities between the target and the
errored output in phonetic features and phonetic environment.
Furthermore, the permissibility of the output as meaningful words of
the same syntactic class as the intended targets also plays a part in
these errors. However, the most revealing characteristic is that they
do not tend to cross phrase boundaries. This suggests that the sound
structure of utterances are constructed phrase by phrase. Not only

might it be useful to examine the nature of such errors to determine their occurrence in disordered children, but it may also reveal something about their knowledge of phrase structures. There are procedures (see, e.g., Dell, 1986) for 'priming' such errors.

Information level and stress

An extremely important aspect of communication is the distinction between new and old information. The distinction manifests itself in many ways. A speaker who is sensitive to the needs of the listener makes certain efforts to adjust the message to the listener's needs. There are also some specific linguistic conventions. We tend to talk about and, given a choice, tend to encode new information. Old information can be pronominalized, referred to using definite articles or omitted (ellipsis) and topicalized. New information can be stressed and serves as the comment in an utterance.

In any situation when a speaker is providing new information to a listener it is logical to expect an effort to ensure that communication is successful. One obvious way to do this is to produce speech differently than one might under circumstances where the information is assumed to be not as new to the listener. Specifically, we might hypothesize that words encoding new information would be produced more accurately than those encoding old information. Several investigations seem to indicate that this factor does affect production characteristics in normally developing children, in speech-disordered children and, most recently, in adults.

One caveat before considering some of these research findings concerns the relationship between stress and information level. New information tends to be accented or stressed relative to old information. As I will discuss below, there is evidence that children produce stressed syllables more accurately than unstressed syllables. It is unclear whether this simply carries over to the old/new distinction or whether there is an added or independent effect.

The interaction between stress and the topic/comment distinction in influencing phonetic accuracy has been demonstrated in the speech of phonologically disordered children (Campbell and Shriberg, 1982). In spontaneous speech these children exhibited fewer errors in producing comments (new information) than topics (old information) and in stressed than unstressed words. The interaction of stress and information level is illustrated by the fact that the children produced stressed comments more accurately than stressed topics. The findings are provocative, but the study involved a very small number of subjects and did not control for information level. In a more recent investigation an experimental paradigm was used to examine the effect of information level on young normal children's phonetic accuracy (Goffman and Schwartz, 1988). In this investigation, children were asked to describe successive triplets of pictures each involving two objects, with the intent of having the child produce noun–noun utterances. For example, a two-triplet sequence might have been presented as: *cup wagon* (new information level), *shoe wagon* (moderate), *girl* (new) *wagon* (old), *girl* (moderate) *candy, girl* (old) *bottle.* This procedure allowed us careful control over information level and other factors. Words representing new information were produced more accurately than those encoding old information. A recent investigation (Fowler and Housum, 1987) involving adults did not reveal a similar effect of information level on accuracy. However, they did find a significant reduction in the duration of words when they were produced for a second time. This reduction also appears to be salient to listeners as a way of distinguishing old and new information. In the course of normal development, then, children must gradually shift from an accuracy effect of information level to a rhythmic (duration and stress or prominence) effect.

Interestingly, few traditional assessment procedures and intervention activities involve the communication of new information. Naming pictures that both the speaker and the listener can see and identify. In an unpublished study, Weiner (personal communication, 1979) compared the results of administering an articulation test in a standard and a referential condition. In the referential condition a barrier was placed between the clinician and the child. The child had a bound version of the test and the clinician had the individual plates/pictures (mixed in random order) from the same test. The child's task was to instruct the clinician to pass the plates through a slot in the barrier, one at a time, in the order in which they appear in the test booklet available to the child. Because the clinician does not know which of the pages the child is looking at, the child's utterance is really communicative. The children performed better in the referential condition than in the standard condition. Although children should be able to perform in a standard test condition, clinical procedures are needed that can tap children's ability to perform under more natural communicative conditions. In intervention, the only methods that really capitalize on information level involve some minimal pair or contrast approaches (e.g. giving a child a picture of a boat and requiring them to ask a clinician for another when the choices are pictures of a *bow* and a *boat*).

Communicative failures can provide a natural situation in which it is clear that the information the speaker will produce is new to the listener. This includes cases in which the listener indicates a lack of understanding by ignoring the speaker, by responding inappropriately, or by requesting clarification (e.g. *What?, Huh?*) and the speaker must respond by repairing the original utterance. This first seems to develop an MLU level of about 1.5 when children first recognize the need to respond to indications of communicative failure. The most common repair at this point in both normal and language-impaired children is a phonetic revision of the original utterance (Gallagher, 1977; Gallagher and Darnton, 1979). Language-impaired children continue to rely on phonetic revisions through more advanced stages of development. In these investigations half of the children's revisions were in the direction of a more accurate production; the other half remained the same, involved a different error or were even less accurate than the original production. Other investigators (see Clark, 1982, for a review) have found that both listener-initiated and self-initiated (without any indication from a listener) phonological repairs are the most frequent category of repair in young normally developing children. In contrast to Gallagher's findings, the majority of phonological repairs tended to be in the direction of the adult target. In our own clinic we have worked with some children on revisions as one way of encouraging more accurate productions. In one instance, a Down Syndrome child was encouraged to respond to requests for clarification. The strategy emphasized was repetition with a revision in rate (slowing down). Although this child was not explicitly taught to make phonetic revisions, he began to do so on his own.

Other situations involving clarification requests yield similar findings. For example, children with multiple speech-sound errors who are asked, 'Did you say _____?' tend to provide responses that are more accurate than their initial productions. The greatest improvement occurred when the examiner made an error that was different from the one made by the child.

As I mentioned earlier, stress may play an important role in the information-level effect. In stress-timed languages (stressed syllables are longer than unstressed syllables) such as English, children seem to have difficulty reducing these syllables as adults do. Instead, they are frequently omitted or produced incorrectly. In addition, there may also be a serial-position effect (see Allen and Hawkins, 1980, for a review), suggesting a trochaic constraint in which children prefer words with falling accent (stressed or prominent first syllables).

Words with unstressed initial syllables would be produced without their initial syllables. In a recent experiment, children's imitative productions of minimal pairs of nonsense words (e.g. *'soti* vs *so'ti*) were examined (Schwartz and Goffman, 1988). The children's tendency to delete syllables was influenced by stress and their segmental accuracy tended to be influenced more by position. Unstressed syllables were most likely to be deleted; first-position syllables were most likely to be produced accurately. The children also produced first-position stressed syllables more accurately than first-position unstressed syllables. In Spanish, the preference for a trochaic pattern seems to depend on the word structure (Hochberg, 1987). Spanish-speaking children make the fewest errors in producing words with final-syllable stress when they end in a consonant. The words with penultimate stress that are produced most accurately are those that end in a vowel. It seems obvious that we have a great deal to learn about the effects of suprasegmental factors in explaining a number of characteristics of children's phonological behaviour, including the effects of information level.

Perception/comprehension

Two aspects of reception can be considered. The first concerns production–perception relationships. Beyond a simplistic tack of trying to determine the developmental or temporal relationship between production and perception/comprehension (i.e., does perception or comprehension precede production? – the answer has usually been yes), we have made only limited strides in understanding these relationships, particularly across language components (see Clark and Hecht, 1983, for a review). It seems possible that there is an initial separation between production and perception representations in a given domain, with only later co-ordination as development proceeds (Schwartz and Leonard, 1982; Clark and Hecht, 1983).

Speech perception can be affected by a number of linguistic factors. Semantic information, word familiarity, word-form class, suprasegmental features can all play an important role in adult's speech perception (e.g. Grosjean and Gee, 1987; Marslen-Wilson, 1987). However, we still actually know very little about the abilities of children under three years of age.

One direction of great interest is the work that reveals a consistent deficit in the perception of brief and rapidly changing acoustic information by children with specific language impairment (see Tallal and Stark, forthcoming). Though it is clearly not the underlying cause of such impairments, it may be one of several related factors including certain motor-speech and non-speech deficits. For example, given these perceptual limitations, difficulties in perceiving unstressed, brief stretches of speech such as grammatical morphemes may have a significant impact on parsing and, consequently, syntactic processing as well as acquisition. These children may also have difficulties recognizing durational cues that distinguish new and old information and identify phrase-structure breaks. At the other end of the spectrum are children, sometimes termed developmentally apraxic, who have apparent motor-speech limitations in the absence of any perceptual limitations.

As better methodologies become available for research and clinical application, we will be able to examine perceptual abilities to determine children's perceptually based knowledge of phonology and its interaction with other aspects of language and with various facets of production.

CONCLUSION

The nature and scope of the interactions among language components are such that it is difficult to imagine an attempt to assess or to remediate a phonological or any other type of language disorder in isolation from other language components. Furthermore, it is possible that what is often characterized as random variability in the behaviour of children may be readily explained by some of these interactions. By modifying assessment and intervention procedures to accommodate these relationships we may enhance the quality of our clinical procedures. By recognizing the significance of individual profiles across language components, we may begin to define a clinically relevant typology of linguistic disorders.

REFERENCES

Allen, G. and Hawkins, S. (1980) 'Phonological rhythm: definition and development', in G. Yeni-Komshian, J. Kavanagh and C. Ferguson (eds) *Child Phonology*, vol. 1: *Production*, New York: Academic Press.

Bock, K. (1982) 'Toward a cognitive psychology of syntax: information processing contributions to sentence formulation', *Psychological Review* 89: 1–47.

Bock, K. (1987a) 'An effect of the accessibility of word forms on sentence structures', *Journal of Memory and Language* 26: 119–37.

Bock, K. (1987b) 'Co-ordinating words and syntax in speech plans', in A.W. Ellis (ed.) *Progress in the Psychology of Language*, vol. 3, London: Lawrence Erlbaum.

Branigan, G. (1976) 'Some reasons why single-word utterances are not', *Journal of Child Language* 6: 411–21.

Camarata, S. and Leonard, L.B. (1986) 'Young children pronounce object words more accurately than action words', *Journal of Child Language* 13: 51–65.

Camarata, S. and Schwartz, R. (1985) 'Production of action words and object words: evidence for a relationship between semantics and phonology', *Journal of Speech and Hearing Research* 28: 323–30.

Campbell, T.F. and Shriberg, L.D. (1982) 'Associations among pragmatic functions, linguistic stress, and natural phonological processes in speech-delayed children', *Journal of Speech and Hearing Research* 25: 547–53.

Clark, E. (1982) 'Language change during language acquisition', in M. Lamb and A. Brown (eds) *Advances in Developmental Psychology*, vol. 2, Hillsdale, NJ: Lawrence Erlbaum, 171–95.

Clark, E. and Hecht, B. (1983) 'Comprehension, production and language acquisition', in M. Rosenzweig (ed.) *Annual Review of Psychology* 34: 325–49

Cohen, G. (1978) 'The effects of linguistic and contextual variables on /s/ productions in children with inconsistent /s/ articulation', unpublished doctoral dissertation, Memphis State University.

Cooper, W. and Sorenson, J. (1981) *Fundamental Frequency in Sentence Production*, New York: Springer.

Crystal, D. (1987) 'Towards a "bucket" theory of language disability: taking account of interaction between linguistic levels', *Clinical Linguistics and Phonetics* 1: 7–22.

Dell, G. (1986) 'A spreading activation theory of retrieval in sentence production', *Psychological Review* 93: 283–321.

DeVilliers, J. and DeVilliers, P. (1978) 'Simplifying phonological processes in the one- and two-word stage', paper presented at the Boston University Conference on Child Language Development, Boston, MA.

Donahue, M. (1986) 'Phonological constraints on the emergence of two-word utterances', *Journal of Child Language* 13: 209–18.

Faircloth, M. and Faircloth, S. (1970) 'An analysis of the articulation behavior of a speech defective child in connected speech and isolated word responses', *Journal of Speech and Hearing Disorders* 35: 51–61.

Ferguson, C. and Farwell, C. (1975) 'Words and sounds in early language acquisition: English initial consonants in the first fifty words', *Language* 51: 419–39.

Fowler, C. and Housum, J. (1987) 'Talkers' signaling of "new" and "old" words in speech and listeners' perception and use of the distinction', *Journal of Memory and Language* 26: 489–504.

Fromkin, V., (ed.) (1973) *Speech Errors as Linguistic Evidence*, The Hague: Mouton.

Gallagher, T. (1977) 'Revision behaviors in the speech of normal children developing language', *Journal of Speech and Hearing Research* 20: 303–18.

Garrett, M. (1980) 'Levels of processing in sentence production', in B.

Butterworth (ed.) *Language Production* vol. 1, London: Academic Press, 177–220.

Goffman, L. and Schwartz, R. (1988) 'Information level and phonetic accuracy in young children', unpublished paper, Purdue University.

Grosjean, F. and Gee, J. (1987) 'Prosodic structure and spoken word recognition', *Cognition* 25: 135–56.

Hochberg, J. (1987) 'The acquisition of word stress rules in Spanish', *Papers and Reports on Child Language Development* 26: 56–63.

Hogg, R. and McCully, C. (1987) *Metrical Phonology: a Coursebook*, Cambridge: Cambridge University Press.

Kamhi, A., Catts, H. and Davis, M. (1984) 'Management of sentence production demands', *Journal of Speech and Hearing Research* 27: 329–38.

Klatt, D. (1975) 'Vowel lengthening is syntactically determined in a connected discourse', *Journal of Phonetics* 3: 129–40.

Leonard, L., Schwartz, R., Loeb, D. and Swanson, L. (1987) 'Some conditions that promote unusual phonological behavior in children', *Clinical Linguistics and Phonetics* 1: 23–34.

Leonard, L., Schwartz, R., Chapman, K., Rowan, L., Prelock, P., Terrell, B., Weiss, A. and Messick, C. (1982) 'Early lexical acquisition in children with specific language impairment', *Journal of Speech and Hearing Research* 25: 554–64.

Marslen-Wilson, W. (1987) 'Functional parallelism in spoken word-recognition', *Cognition* 25: 71–102.

Masterson, J. and Kamhi, A. (1985) 'Linguistic and extralinguistic influences upon children's sentence productions', paper presented at the American Speech-Language-Hearing Convention, Washington.

Messick, C. (1984) 'Phonetic and contextual aspects of the transition to early words', unpublished doctoral dissertation, Purdue University, West Lafayette, IN.

Messick, C. and Schwartz, R. (1982) 'Does imitation or comprehension affect phonological production in Stage I children?', paper presented to the American Speech, Language and Hearing Association, Toronto.

Nelson, L. and Kamhi, A. (1984) 'Syntactic, semantic and phonological trade-offs in preschool children's utterances', paper presented to the American Speech, Language and Hearing Association, San Francisco.

Panagos, J. (1974) 'Persistence of the open syllable reinterpreted as a symptom of language disorder', *Journal of Speech and Hearing Disorders* 39: 23–31.

Panagos, J. (1982) 'The case against the autonomy of phonological disorders in children', *Seminars in Speech, Language, and Hearing* 3: 172–82.

Paul, R. and Shriberg, L. (1982) 'Associations between phonology and syntax in speech-delayed children', *Journal of Speech and Hearing Research* 25: 536–47.

Prelock, P. (1983) 'Cumulative effects of syntactic and phonological complexity on children's language production', unpublished doctoral dissertation, University of Pittsburgh.

Schwartz, R. (1988) 'Phonological factors in early lexical acquisition', in M. Smith and J. Locke (eds) *The Emergent Lexicon: the Child's Development of a Linguistic Vocabulary*, San Diego: Academic Press, 185–224.

Schwartz, R. and Goffman, L. (1988) 'The effect of syllabic stress and word position on production accuracy', submitted to *Journal of Child Language.*

Schwartz, R. and Leonard, L. (1982) 'Do children pick and choose? An examination of phonological selection and avoidance in early lexical acquisition', *Journal of Child Language* 9: 319–36.

Schwartz, R., Messick, C. and Pollock, K. (1983) 'some non-phonological considerations in phonological assessment', in J. Locke (ed.) *Seminars in Speech and Language*, vol. 4, no. 4, 335–49.

Schwartz, R., Leonard, L., Folger, M. and Wilcox, M. (1980) 'Evidence for a linguistic view of phonological disorder: early phonological behavior in normal and language disordered children', *Journal of Speech and Hearing Disorders* 45: 357–77.

Schwartz, R., Leonard, L., Loeb, D. and Swanson, L. (1987) 'Attempted sounds are sometimes not: an expanded view of phonological selection and avoidance', *Journal of Child Language* 14: 411–18.

Selkirk, E. (1984) *Phonology and Syntax: the Relation between Sound and Structure*, Cambridge, MA: MIT Press.

Sorenson, J., Cooper, W. and Paccia, J. (1978) 'Speech timing of grammatical categories', *Cognition* 6: 135–53.

Stemberger, J.P. (1985) 'An interactive activation model of language production', in A.W. Ellis (ed.) *Progress in the Psychology of Language*, vol. 1, London: Erlbaum.

Stemberger, J.P. (1988) 'Between-word processes in child phonology', *Journal of Child Language* 15: 39–62.

Stoel-Gammon, C. and Cooper, J. (1984) 'Patterns of early lexical and phonological development', *Journal of Child Language* 11: 247–71.

Waterson, N. (1978) 'Growth of complexity in phonological development', in N. Waterson and C. Snow (eds) *The Development of Communication*, Chichester: Wiley.

Weiner, F. and Ostrowski, A. (1979) 'Effects of listener uncertainty on articulatory inconsistency', *Journal of Speech and Hearing Disorders* 44: 487–93.

4 Metalinguistic awareness in phonologically disordered children

Eva Magnusson

During the last ten to fifteen years there has been a growing interest in linguistic awareness among linguists, psycholinguists, psychologists and educators. This has been the impetus for a lot of research about linguistic awareness in children with a normal language acquisition.

The interest in, and the accumulating amount of data about, linguistic awareness in normal children has no real equivalent so far in information about linguistic awareness in language-disordered children. Until recently, clinicians and researchers with an interest in speech and language pathology have to a large extent ignored the topic, either because it has not been considered relevant or as a consequence of the often observed delay in applying new ideas and approaches from other disciplines, such as linguistics and psychology, to the study of language pathology and to the development of intervention strategies.

Knowledge about children's ability to reflect upon language can contribute to our understanding of phonological disorders and to our handling of such problems in clinical and educational practice. Ideas about how and why children become aware of language are relevant in this connection as well as the role that is attributed to linguistic awareness in child development.

DEVELOPMENT OF METALINGUISTIC AWARENESS

Different opinions have been put forward about the development and functions of linguistic awareness, suggesting a close relationship with either language acquisition, cognitive development, or the acquisition of literacy.

Among researchers who advocate a close link between linguistic awareness and language acquisition there are different opinions about how linguistic awareness is related to the acquisition of language. The different views go back to the role of conscious cognition in the acquisition of a new skill. According to one view, we are most aware of a skill at the time when we are acquiring it and, consequently, children would be linguistically aware from the early stages of language acquisition (Clark, 1978; Marshall and Morton, 1978).

An opposing view about the relation between linguistic awareness and language acquisition is held by those who claim that we cannot be aware of a skill until it is acquired (Vygotsky, 1962). Consequently, children would not become aware of language until they have acquired it. Linguistic awareness is seen as a further development of linguistic abilities beyond what is needed for speech perception and production. This type of reasoning would predict phonologically disordered children to be less linguistically aware than normally developing children as a consequence of their deficient linguistic knowledge and, furthermore, that linguistic awareness would not emerge in disordered children until they have overcome their linguistic difficulties.

According to another way of thinking, linguistic awareness is closely tied to cognitive development and reflects the change in cognitive functioning that is observed in children during middle childhood, approximately from four to eight years of age (e.g. Sinclair, 1978). The child proceeds from the preoperational stage to the concrete-operational period, to use Piagetian terms. This change in cognitive functioning is reflected both in later language development and in the emergence of linguistic awareness. Experimental evidence for a relation between performance on Piagetian conservation tasks and linguistic awareness has been put forward by Hakes (1980). The child becomes able to 'decentre', to control the course of his or her own thoughts. Language is not just embedded in meaning, as for the preoperational child, but can be made an object of thought; words can be separated from their referents and structural features can be focused on instead of only being used to convey meaning. This new attitude to mental processes is not restricted to language but can be noticed in all cognitive processes. According to this view linguistic awareness is one way in which the newly acquired metacognitive capacity of the concrete-operational child is evident.

If linguistic awareness is just one of several ways in which the change in cognitive functioning during middle childhood is reflected, we would predict no differences in the ability to reflect upon language in children developing language normally and in phonologically disordered children as long as their cognitive developmental level is the same.

The third view links linguistic awareness to the acquisition of language in its written form. A correlation between linguistic awareness and reading has been reported in a lot of studies, showing good readers and spellers to be linguistically aware and poor readers and spellers to be unaware (for a review see Bertelson, 1986). This has led some researchers to consider linguistic awareness as resulting from reading instruction and the acquisition of reading (e.g. Valtin, 1984), while others see linguistic awareness as a prerequisite for learning to read and write (e.g. Liberman *et al.*, 1977). An intermediate position is taken by those who hold an interactive view, i.e. that certain aspects of linguistic awareness are prerequisites for learning to read and write, while others result from the acquisition of literacy (Ehri, 1984: Morais *et al.*, 1987). The relationship between linguistic awareness and reading is of special interest in connection with phonologically disordered children, as we know that a majority of the phonologically disordered children, but not all of them, have problems learning to read and write, and that this is the case even if they have normalized their speech before starting school.

The ages that are mentioned for the emergence of linguistic awareness in normal children differ widely. Some find evidence for the emergence of linguistic awareness before children are two years old (e.g. Clark, 1978). Spontaneous self-repairs, corrections of others, adjustment of speech in social situations and to different listeners as well as verbal play, as described by Weir (1962) in her son's bedtime monologues where structural features are systematically varied and practised, are cited as early signs of linguistic awareness. According to Clark repairs play an important role in children's acquisition of language from the early stages. Repairs are seen as indicative of children's abilities to monitor and check their own utterances, leading to a realization that their language is inadequate. This insight is assumed to motivate children to change their language. Other researchers do not report children to be metalinguistically aware until the age of six or seven, when children become able, e.g., to make phonemic segmentation (Nesdale *et al.*, 1984). This variation of age is due to the kind of evidence that different researchers are willing to accept as reflections of children's awareness of language which in turn is dependent on how linguistic awareness is defined.

DEFINING METALINGUISTIC AWARENESS

There is some controversy as to what behaviours are to be considered as evidence for linguistic awareness. Repairs, for instance, are seen as attempts to repair communicative failures where the communicative break-down forces the child to pay attention to why his or her utterance did not convey the intended meaning. Some hold the view that this forces the child to reflect upon linguistic structure and linguistic features in order to repair inadequate utterances (Clark, 1978), while others want to make a clear distinction between awareness of communicative failure and awareness of linguistic structure (Tunmer and Herriman, 1984). Young children are aware of the goal they want to achieve, the intended meaning of their utterances, and are aware of their failures to convey their intended meaning. This certainly goes for phonologically disordered children as well. Awareness of failure leads the children to make a new attempt to convey their meaning, but this does not necessarily mean that they have considered linguistic structure and made conscious manipulations of linguistic forms in order to get their meaning across.

Children interacting verbally with persons in a social context are concerned with making themselves understood, not with linguistic form and structure. Children who are linguistically competent, who are able to perceive and produce language forms, are not necessarily aware of the linguistic forms they use to convey meaning. Only when there is clear evidence that children disregard content and reflect upon, make explicit comments about or consciously manipulate linguistic forms and features are we justified in claiming that they are linguistically aware.

Several suggestions have been made about how to define linguistic awareness, focusing on either linguistic or psychological aspects of the concept. One of the first to use the term linguistic awareness was Mattingly (1972) who used it to describe the speaker's/listener's conscious reflections or insights about certain aspects of primary linguistic activities such as speaking and listening rather than the activity itself. Later, Mattingly defines linguistic awareness as a person's access to his or her knowledge of the grammatical structure of sentences. Grammatical knowledge is intuitive knowledge and hence accessible, while the strategies to use such knowledge, e.g. in speech perception and production, are inaccessible.

In psychologically orientated definitions linguistic awareness is seen as reflecting a change in cognitive functioning, allowing refection upon the products of mental operations. The ability to make language an object of thought is considered as one of the metacognitive skills that follows from the concrete-operational child's ability to decentre. This has been expressed as an attention shift from content to form, 'an ability to make language forms opaque and attend to them in and for themselves' (Cazden 1976: 603) by invoking Luria's glass-window theory. Attention may be shifted from what is seen through the window to the glass itself, from meaning to language that is used to convey this meaning.

Whatever definition we adopt, it is often problematic to draw a sharp line between linguistic awareness and other related areas. Van Kleeck (1984a), among others, points to the difficulty in making a strict distinction between linguistic awareness and pragmatics, defined as the practical skill of using language in social contexts, on one hand, and metacognition, defined as insight regarding cognitive processes, on the other. A certain amount of overlapping is at hand here, while there is a sharp demarcation line towards metacommunication which is the term used for non-linguistic means to convey messages, e.g. facial expressions, gestures, uses of distance and space, clothing are considered part of pragmatics. Metapragmatics, reflections on social rules of language use and comments on what is a socially acceptable way of talking in a given situation, is also seen as distinct from linguistic awareness. Pratt and Nesdale (1984), on the other hand, regard pragmatic awareness as one aspect of linguistic awareness, although they remark that 'it incorporates aspects that extend beyond linguistic considerations' (p. 105). They define pragmatic awareness as

> awareness or knowledge one has about the relationships that obtain within the linguistic system itself (e.g. across different sentences) and with the relationships that obtain between the linguistic system and the context in which language is embedded (e.g. speaker's ability to match his utterance to suit the listener's previous knowledge and current perspective)
>
> (Pratt and Nesdale, 1984: 105)

STUDIES OF METALINGUISTIC AWARENESS IN DISORDERED CHILDREN

In the following discussion we will primarily be concerned with phonological aspects of children's ability to reflect upon language. This is the area where most of the work on disordered children has been done and it also seems the most relevant aspect in connection with phonologically disordered children. We will start by discussing what is known about disordered children's awareness of words, syllables and phonemes. In the section on clinical implications some work on syntactic awareness will be included as well as examples of studies of pragmatic awareness, although there is some controversy as to its status, whether or not to consider it part of linguistic awareness. Despite their doubtful status, some such studies are referred to because of their clinical implications. In reviewing the research on linguistic awareness in phonologically disordered children, special attention will be paid to the type of task that is used to measure linguistic awareness and to the demands they make on other abilities. This will be done with the aim of evaluating how well suited they are to the special requirements on tests to be used with phonologically disordered children.

As in the study of linguistic awareness in normal children most of the research regarding phonologically disordered children has been undertaken by researchers interested in reading and writing, either in attempts to predict reading and writing achievements or to study the relation between linguistic awareness and reading and writing proficiency. In studies of language-disordered children's reading and spelling, tests of linguistic awareness are mentioned among other tests of background factors. In most studies the language-disordered children are compared to normally speaking children or to groups of reading-impaired children who have no history of language disorder. Very few papers are concerned with linguistic awareness without making references to its role in reading and writing. The research done on poor readers will not be included here, even if we know that a lot of the poor readers have a history of language disorders, and there is some overlapping between the two populations. The data from studies of poor readers are considered rather off the point when discussing linguistic awareness in phonologically disordered children, as we know that all poor readers have not have developmental language problems and all language-disordered children will not have reading and writing problems.

Except for papers reporting experimental evidence for linguistic awareness in disordered children, there are observations mentioned in passing scattered through the language-pathology literature but no investigation of spontaneous examples of linguistic awareness in disordered children, e.g. of spontaneous repairs, corrections of others, language play. Some discussion about clinical implications has been initiated (e.g. Van Kleeck, 1984b; Dean and Howell, 1986).

Word awareness

In order to manipulate or make judgements about linguistic structures, children have to be able to disregard content and to focus on the linguistic form, thereby showing an awareness of words as distinct from what they refer to and of language as an arbitrary conventional code. One type of evidence for this is children's ability to realize that a word may be short even if it refers to a long object and long even if it refers to something short (e.g. that *train* is a short word and *butterfly* a long one irrespective of the size of their referents). This has been tested by asking children whether words are long or short, taking care to select the words so that word length and referent length or size do not always coincide. This was one of the tasks used in a study by Lagergren and Larsson (1986) of 28 phonologically disordered Swedish children, 12 five-year-olds and 16 six-year-olds. All the children had more or less serious phonological problems and children with more serious phonological impairments also showed other linguistic problems. When word length and referent size were not congruent, the number of correct responses was 53 per cent, as against 83 per cent when they were congruent, indicating some ability to judge word length as distinct from physical characteristics of the referent.

A somewhat different design to study awareness of words was used in a study by Kamhi *et al.* (1985) of fifteen language-impaired children in age from 3;0 to 6;0. These children were matched to fifteen normally developing children on the basis of mental age (MA) and to another fifteen on the basis of language age (LA). Among other tasks in the test battery (see below) there was one task designed to measure word awareness, based on the procedure used by Papandropoulou and Sinclair (1974). The children were asked 'What is a word?', 'Say a long/short word', 'A hard/easy word' and 'What makes words long, short?', etc. The language-disordered children could not make any distinction between words and their referents, e.g. as an answer to the question 'What is a word?', they gave examples such as *table* or *ball* instead of a definition. They tried to answer some of the questions but their answers did not make sense. The LA- and MA-matched children realized that words are used to refer to something, although they only considered content words as words, not function words. Only two of the MA-matched children realized that words are distinct from what they refer to and could give sensible answers to some of the questions about long and short words.

The disordered children in the Kamhi *et al.* study do not appear to be aware of words, while the children in the Lagergren and Larsson study seem to have some ideas about long and short words. It is to be noted that the tasks are different. In the Swedish study the children had to decide whether a word is long or short, to choose between two alternatives, while the task in the other study made demands of another and more advanced nature. Beside defining the meta-linguistic term *word*, the children were expected to give examples of long and short words and to tell what makes these words long or short. It is not unreasonable to assume that children may be aware of words as phonological or lexical units without knowing the meta-linguistic term for these units. In this case they would not to able to give a definition of the term *word*, but they would be able to perform tasks that reflect an awareness of words, e.g. dividing sentences into words. Depending on the difference between the tasks, the children in one study appeared to be able to judge the length of words, separate from the size of the referent, while children of approximately the same age in the other study were not able to do so. In the study by Kamhi *et al.*, three- and four-year-old children were included, beside the five- and six-year-olds, but the fact that younger children are included cannot explain that none of the children in this study showed any awareness of words. As we will see in the following, the type of task is an important factor to keep in mind when evaluating results from different tests developed to measure the same ability, and is a factor that may explain conflicting results.

The task in the Kamhi *et al.* study, where the children have to define metalinguistic terms and give verbal explanations instead of making a choice between two alternatives, is to the language-disordered children's disadvantage. In studies of linguistic awareness in disordered children, there is a risk that their linguistic disability may prevent them from giving evidence of their ability to reflect upon language if a response type is chosen that makes high demands on verbal ability. Their difficulties in using language to express their ideas may be mistaken for lack of awareness.

This disadvantage is eliminated if word awareness is tested by having children divide sentences into words. This task has been used together with other segmentation tasks in the earlier mentioned study by Kamhi *et al.* (1985) and by Kamhi and Catts (1986). In both studies the same type of segmentation task was used, developed from the procedure described by Fox and Routh (1975), but with linguistic structures somewhat simplified in order to be within the linguistic abilities of the language-impaired children. The task was to divide sentences into words by saying a little of the sentence at a time. If the children gave a multiword phrase, they were again asked to say a little of that until they had divided it into separate words. The sentences varied in length, from two to seven words, and in order to ensure that they did not exceed the short-term memory limits of the children, they were asked to repeat the sentences before doing the segmentation. Scores were given for the number of divisions made.

In the first of these two studies, fewer than 50 per cent of the language-impaired children, in the ages 3;0 to 6;0, managed the task, while 70 per cent of the younger LA-matched children and all the MA-matched children could do it. When these results are compared to the earlier mentioned results on the word-awareness task, given to the same children, where they had to define the term *word* and to give examples of words, we find that about half of the disordered children showed an awareness of words by dividing sentences into words, while none of them showed the kind of awareness that is required in order to give a definition.

In the second study twelve language-impaired children in the ages 6;2 to 9;2 years were compared to twelve reading-impaired children with no history of language disorders and to twelve normal children with the primary purpose of comparing language-impaired and reading-impaired children's ability to process (i.e. to encode and retrieve) phonological information. The word-segmentation task used was managed better by the older children than by the younger ones in the earlier study, thus indicating that linguistic awareness develops also in language-disordered children as they grow older.

Syllable and morpheme awareness

Phonologically disordered children, like normally developing children, seem to be able to segment words at the level of the syllable before they are able to do the same operation at the level of the phoneme. The most widely used syllable-segmentation task in studies of phonologically disordered children is modelled on the procedure described by Liberman *et al.* (1977), where the children indicate the number of syllables in a word by tapping or clapping their hands (Magnusson and Nauclér, 1985, 1987; Lagergren and Larsson, 1986; Snowling, *et al.*, 1986). The words may be varied in a more or less systematic way as to the number of syllables and to stress pattern, the stressed syllable being the first, the second, the third, etc. Five- and six-year-olds made 47 per cent and 57 per cent correct responses respectively on the syllable-segmentation task (Lagergren and Larsson, 1986), which is in agreement with the results in a longitudinal study by Magnusson and Nauclér (1987) of thirty-seven language-disordered children and a matched group of normally developing children from the age of six until eight years, i.e. during a period of two years, from the last preschool year until the end of first grade. The number of children who gave at least 80 per cent correct responses, increased from 11 out of 37 at the age of six to 22 nearly two years after, at the end of grade 1. The performance had also improved for those who did not reach the level of 80 per cent correct. Older disordered children seem to be able to make syllable segmentations, as e.g. three dyslexics in the ages 8;5 to 13;11 who had received speech therapy before starting school and who still had 'articulation difficulties' (Snowling *et al.*, 1986). Whenever comparisons are made with normally developing children it turns out that the disordered children as a group perform less well than groups of normal children (Lagergren and Larsson, 1986; Magnusson and Nauclér, 1987).

A different way of measuring syllable awareness is the one used by Kamhi *et al.* (1985) and by Kamhi and Catts (1986) in the earlier mentioned studies. In a modified version of the procedure described by Fox and Routh (1975), the subjects are asked to say little bits of bisyllabic words where at least one of the segmented parts is always a real word (e.g. *airplane, pencil*). Here again we find that performance is better with older children, but at all comparisons with normal children the disordered group manages less well. For both the disordered children and the normal ones, the segmentation of bisyllabic words into syllables was easier than the segmentation of sentences into words.

In the syllable-segmentation task where the children indicate the number of syllables by tapping or clapping their hands, the segmentations are made with reference only to the sound structure of the words, possibly helped by the acoustic information in the signal (intensity maxima corresponding to the vowels of the syllables). The other procedure where children say a little bit of a bisyllabic word, and at least one syllable is a real word, could be performed in two ways: either at the phonological level by segmentation of the sound structure; or at the semantic/lexical level so that the segmentation task is not purely one of separating syllables at the phonetic/phonological level but could also be undertaken by isolating words or morphemes.

Tasks that explicitly require children to segment words (compound words) into morphemes were given by Lagergren and Larsson (1986) together with a syllable-segmentation task where responses were made by hand clapping. Morphemes resulting from the segmentation of compounds did not always correspond to syllables since bisyllabic morphemes were included. It is interesting to note that the morpheme-segmentation was much more difficult than the syllable-segmentation task, e.g. only 2 per cent of the five-year-old children's responses on the morpheme-segmentation task was correct compared to 47 per cent on the syllable-segmentation task. Besides the fact that the segmentations may be performed on different linguistic levels, the syllables task only requires an indication of the number of syllables, whereas in the morpheme-segmentation task it is not only a question of the number of parts but of identifying the parts, as the children were to indicate what was left of a word if part of it was taken away.

If the language-disordered children's performance on these two tasks is compared to that of normal children, we find that the difference in how the tasks are managed, is larger for the disordered children than for the normal ones as a consequence of the disordered children's comparatively larger problems with morpheme segmentation. The syllable-segmentation task, where easily accessible acoustic information may help the decisions, is managed comparatively better than the morpheme-segmentation task, where the disordered children may be at a disadvantage for two reasons: because their lexicons are restricted and/or because the lexical information is less easily accessible.

It can be mentioned that synthetization of morphemes (yielding compounds like *airplane* from *air* and *plane*) is easier than the segmentation of compounds into morphemes. In the Lagergren and Larsson study this is so for both five- and six-year-olds, who made 35 per cent and 69 per cent correct responses respectively, and for the normal children who made 54 per cent and 83 per cent correct responses. A possible explanation for the difference between synthetization and segmentation could be that the synthetization of auditorily presented morphemes could be performed at a phonological level, by minimizing the pause between the items. The segmentation, on the other hand, cannot be done without the ability of alternating between the phonological and the semantic/lexical level. The phonological form of the word has to be used for the segmentation and where the delimitations are to be made, cannot be decided without reference to the semantic level. If the children cannot take the phonological form as their starting point, they end up trying to take qualities or attributes away from the referent so that the answer to the question 'What is left of *crocodile* if *croco* is taken away?' may be 'The tail'. What is needed is an ability to be simultaneously aware of more than one linguistic level.

To be aware of several linguistic levels at the same time is one of the requirements for the appreciation of jokes, puns and riddles. This is a relatively late acquisition for normal children which is not fully developed until the age of ten or eleven (Hirsch-Pasek *et al.*, 1978) and a pleasure that may not be discovered at all by disordered children. In order to appreciate jokes involving, for instance, homophones and ambiguities, phonological awareness is considered important as well as the simultaneous awareness of more than one linguistic level. Clinicians working with phonologically disordered children often notice that many of the disordered children do not seem to appreciate verbal jokes and ambiguities (Van Kleeck, 1984b).

Phoneme awareness

Phoneme awareness is the aspect of phonological awareness that has been most thoroughly investigated in phonologically disordered children. Various tasks have been used that differ considerably both as to the level of phoneme awareness that is required to manage them and as to the type of demands on other skills that are made by the particular task. In some only partial segmentation is required, while a complete segmentation and identification of the elements in the phoneme sequence are needed for the completion of others.

One way of studying phoneme awareness is to look at children's rhyming ability. In order to understand the rhyming principle and to invent rhymes children have to be able to shift their attention from the meaning of words to their structural form. Furthermore, they have to be aware of the possibility of segmenting words and syllables into smaller units. They have to be able to separate any prevocalic consonant(s) in the stressed syllable from the vowel and the following consonant(s) and to use what is left of the syllable after the separation as a model when producing new rhymes. Rhyming thus requires the ability to make segmentation within the syllable, although a complete segmentation and identification of all the phonemes in the sequence is not needed. Beside the segmentation, a categorization of the relevant parts of words as identical or not identical is also needed.

In most studies of disordered children's rhyming, some type of rhyme-detection task has been used. By this procedure the risk is minimized that the task will not be managed because of the disordered children's limited lexicons. Phonologically disordered children asked to produce spontaneous rhymes may demonstrate their understanding of the rhyming principle by giving one rhyming word but then go on to give semantically related words or quite unrelated ones or to make alliterations (Stackhouse and Snowling, 1983; Stackhouse, 1985). One child, mentioned by Stackhouse, at the age of 10 years and 7 months gave the following suggestions for words rhyming with the target *map*: *train, map, trap, hatch, mat, mop*. Semantic associations are made by normal children before they are able to rhyme, around the age of three, but may be the only strategy at hand for language-disordered children in their teens (Stackhouse, 1985). Also, adults, who have a history of serious language disorders in childhood, have been observed to prefer a semantic rhyming strategy (Nauclér, personal communication).

If children fail to produce a rhyming word, we do not know if it is because they do not understand the rhyming concept or because they find no words in their lexicon with the required sound structure. Disordered children do not suggest nonsense words in this situation, as normal children are likely to do and enjoy doing, which is quite in line with phonologically disordered children's reluctance to deal with nonsense words in any situation. A possible explanation is that the phonologically disordered children do not have effective phonological coding strategies and have to rely more heavily than normal children on semantic coding instead of on a phonological representation. In cases where only a phonological coding strategy works and no semantic coding is possible, for instance in the repetition of nonsense words, the disordered children cannot cope.

For these reasons it seems advisable to use some type of rhyme-detection or rhyme-judgement task in studies of language-disordered children's rhyming. This was the procedure used in a study by Magnusson (1983) of twenty-seven phonologically disordered children in the ages 3;9 to 6;6. The children were shown three pictures which were named during conversation, and the children's task was to indicate the two rhyming words in the triplet by pointing to the pictures. The third word was a distractor with either a strong semantic association with one of the rhyming words or identical prevocalic consonants, thus making semantic choices and alliteration possible. The children were instructed to respond by pointing, instead of saying the words, in order to avoid any uncertainties in the analysis of their responses due to their deviant speech production. Ten of the children were classed as good rhymers, while another five were considered as poor rhymers, i.e. they were on their way to mastering the task, and twelve were classed as non-rhymers.

In the non-rhyming group, the erroneous choices appeared to be random or based on semantic associations, which is the type of choice we would expect from children who are not able to disregard content and focus on the linguistic expression. The erroneous choices made by the poor rhymers (and by the good rhymers, if they made any) were alliterations, thus showing that their choices were based on considerations of the sound structure of the words even if they compared the beginnings of words instead of the ends. Alliteration responses are explained by Stackhouse and Snowling (1983) as a possible teaching effect resulting from speech therapy and/or phonic training in the course of reading instruction. Bradley and Bryant (1985) make a similar suggestion about the effect of reading instruction for normal children. This explanation does not hold for the alliterations made by the disordered children in this study, as none of the children had had speech therapy or been subject to reading instruction at the time of the testing. Nor could any of them read. As alliterations were mainly made by the children who also showed at least some grasp of the rhyming principle, and not by non-rhyming children, a more plausible explanation for these observations is that alliterations are made by children who are in the process of discovering rhyme. They are able to disregard content and pay attention only to the form. Furthermore, they have realized that syllables can be segmented into smaller parts, but they are not yet sure which part of the sequence to pay attention to after the segmentation.

No relation was found in this study between age and rhyming ability. Between rhyming and the degree of phonological deviance, there was a weak tendency towards a negative correlation, so that children with a very deviant speech production were more likely to be non-rhymers than children with nearly normal speech. At the same time there were nearly normally speaking children who could not rhyme, and some very deviantly speaking children who were good rhymers, which shows that normal speech is not required for children in order to become rhymers and that an ability to rhyme does not automatically follow from normal speech.

That rhyming without normal speech is possible, is also shown in the case of Genie, a girl with very deviant speech who was able to detect rhymes (Curtiss, 1977) and by the fact that deaf children are able to rhyme (Dodd and Hermelin, 1977). Nor is normal speech a guarantee for the development of rhyming, as shown by the fact that all normally developing children are not able to rhyme. That is it not possible to predict the rhyming ability from the degree of phonological deviance as it is evidenced in speech production is also pointed out by Stackhouse (1985), who states that 'the severity of the speech problem is not necessarily indicative of the severity of the segmentation difficulties' (p. 104).

The same rhyming test was used on twenty-five of the children from the earlier investigation in a follow-up study six years later, when the children were in the ages 10 to 12;6 (Nauclér and Magnusson, 1985). All the children had improved their rhyming ability but there were still four children who did not qualify as rhymers.

In the rhyming task described above, there is a certain cognitive load and high demands are made on memory. The children have to choose one of the three words as a model to which the other two are to be compared. If none of the alternatives is found to be a rhyme, a new model has to be chosen and the comparison gone through again. The demands are less heavy in procedures where one word is given as a target word, and the children's task is to select the rhyming word from two alternatives, one which is a rhyme of the target and the other either semantically related to the target or an alliteration (Stackhouse and Snowling, 1983; Stackhouse, 1985). The rhyme-detection task developed by Bradley and Bryant (1985), and widely used with normal children, where the task is to pick the odd one out in a series of four auditorily presented words where three rhyme and one does not, seems to make too heavy a demand on memory to be used with language-disordered children, who often have a limited short-term memory, at least for verbal material.

In order to alleviate further the cognitive load and the demands on memory, Magnusson *et al.* (1984) developed a rhyming test, partly based on the procedure used by Calfee *et al.* (1980) and modified for use with language-disordered children. The test consists of two parts. In the first part the task is to decide which of three model words, represented by pictures, a test word rhymes with and to indicate the choice by pointing to the picture. The words are selected in such a way that only the test words (CVC structures), and not the models (VC structures), have to be segmented. The vowels in the models are phonetically well separated. In the second part higher demands are made on the children's segmentation ability as well as on their ability to categorize and to discriminate between phonetically close segments. The children are given the model words auditorily and their task is to decide whether or not a number of test words rhyme with the model. The non-rhyming words are varied in such a way that either the vowel or the postvocalic consonant differ from that of the model word, some by several distinctive features and others by only one feature.

This test has been used in two studies of language-disordered and normally speaking children's rhyming abilities, by Magnusson *et al.* (1984) to study ten language-disordered and ten normal children and by Magnusson and Nauclér (1985, 1987) to study seventy-eight language-disordered and thirty-seven normally speaking six-year-old preschool children. In comparisons of the different groups, it was found that the language-disordered children were not as good rhymers as the normal children but, even so, the language-disordered schoolchildren in the first study (aged from 7;1 to 7;10) were better rhymers than the normally developing preschool children (aged from 3;11 to 5;8). The language-disordered six-year-olds in the second study gave 75 per cent correct responses.

All subjects made more mistakes in the second part of the test than in the first one. Several factors may contribute to making the second part more difficult. To decide whether or not pairs of words rhyme, instead of matching a test word to one of three alternatives, seems to be a more demanding task. Observations made by Snowling *et al.* (1986) point in this direction. Their subjects, who had demonstrated that they understood the concept of rhyme, all had difficulties in deciding whether or not word pairs rhymed.

Structural characteristics of the test items also contribute to the differences between the first and the second part of the test. While the task in the first part can be managed by comparing vowels that are phonetically well separated, the second part puts higher demands on both segmentation ability and ability to discriminate between phonetically close segments. Not only does the second part require a more complete segmentation of the phonemic sequence but it also requires the postvocalic consonant(s) to be separated from the vowel, and not only the prevocalic consonant(s) from the rest of the syllable, which is an easier task, as shown by Treiman (1983). This can be interpreted as reflecting the hierarchical structure of the syllable, divisible into onset and rhyme and the rhyme further into peak and coda (Fudge, 1969). In other words, segmentation within the rhyme of the syllable is required and not just a separation of the more loosely attached onset of the syllable from the rhyme. Segmentation within different parts of the syllable is a factor that contributes to the difficulty for all subjects, irrespective of group.

The higher demands on discrimination of phonetically close segments seem more troublesome for language-disordered children than for normal ones. In an analysis of the two types of error that can be made in the second part, false acceptances and false rejections, it was found that children who made relatively few errors in the first part, thereby showing some understanding of the rhyming principle, mainly made false acceptances in the second part. This is seen as an effect of their wider sound categories and discrimination difficulties, an interpretation which seems reasonable as most of the children who showed this pattern were language-disordered. Here we probably have to do with phonologically disordered children who understand the rhyming concept, but who fail on some of the items in the rhyming test because of discrimination difficulties. Corroboration for such a background to some phonologically disordered children's incorrect responses on rhyming tests, comes from the earlier mentioned study of twenty-seven language-disordered children's rhyming (Magnusson, 1983). A group of poor rhymers, children who demonstrated some understanding of rhyming, turned out to consist of the children who had most problems in making auditory discrimination between minimal word pairs.

Rhyming, as we have shown, is a multifaceted task which, among other things, requires an ability to segment within the syllable, although it may be managed without complete segmentation and identification of all the segments in the phonemic sequence. When rhyming tasks are given with other tests designed to measure phonemic awareness, it is more easily managed than phoneme-segmentation and phoneme-identification tasks. In the earlier mentioned studies by Magnusson and Nauclér (1985, 1987) of thirty-seven language-disordered children and a matched group of thirty-seven normally speaking children the following tasks were given in order to measure phonemic awareness in six-year-old preschool children: rhyming, phoneme identification and phoneme segmentation. In the phoneme-identification task the children were asked whether or not a target vowel or consonant was part of a number of words. The target sound appeared in initial, medial or final position of the words. The phoneme-segmentation task was a modified version of the procedure used by Liberman *et al.* (1977) requiring the children to indicate the number of phonemes in words, varied as to length and syllabic structure, by selecting the correct number of markers of some kind. Rhyming turned out to be the easiest task, with 75 per cent correct responses, followed by identification with 66 per cent correct responses. On the segmentation task less than 40 per cent of the responses were correct.

The phoneme-identification and -segmentation tasks, as well as the syllable-segmentation task mentioned earlier, were repeated one year later, right at the beginning of the first school year, and again at the end of the first grade. The children's performance improved on all tasks between each testing. The largest increase was observed during the first school year and concerned the tasks designed to measure phoneme awareness, i.e. the identification and segmentation of phonemes.

The same type of phoneme-segmentation task was used in the earlier mentioned study by Kamhi and Catts (1986) together with two other tasks designed to measure phoneme awareness, a sound-division task modelled on Fox and Routh (1975), also used by Kamhi *et al.* (1985), and an elision task based on Bruce (1964).

In the segmentation task the children were asked to indicate the number of phonemes in a word by tapping. None of the children, aged 6;2 to 9;2, in any group, not even in the normal one, performed better than chance, a result to be compared with those given by Liberman *et al.* (1977) where 70 per cent of normal six-year-olds managed the task, and with results from the Magnusson and Nauclér study (1987) where two out of thirty-seven language-disordered preschool children and six out of thirty-seven normal children managed at least 80 per cent of the items.

The easiest of the other two tasks was the sound-division task. The children were asked to say just a little bit of monosyllabic words and were given an example 'If I say "boat", you could say "boa".' The responses were scored as plus or minus for whether or not the children could segment syllables into smaller units and no scores were given for the number of divisions. This task had been used in an earlier study as well (Kamhi *et al.*, 1985) where only two out of fifteen language-impaired children, aged 3;0 to 6;0, managed the task, while eight of the LA-matched and twelve of the MA-matched children did.

Besides the division of monosyllabic words into sounds, the children were given an elision task. The elision task was the one used by Bruce (1964), where the children are asked to take away a sound from a target word and to indicate what word is left after that manipulation. The sound to be deleted appeared in either initial or final position of the word, e.g. '*t*' was to be taken away in *(t)all* or *ten(t)*. On both these segmentation tasks the children showed a lower degree of phonological awareness than on the previously described one where they said just a little of a word. This draws attention to an important point when evaluating results from tasks designed to measure linguistic awareness: even if the tasks are developed in order to give information about the same aspect of linguistic awareness, e.g. phoneme awareness, the level of awareness seems to differ in the same children depending on which type of task has been used.

The spoonerism task, described by Perin (1983), is another example of a more demanding segmentation task that has been used with phonologically disordered children (Stackhouse, 1985). Here the children are asked to switch the initial phonemes in two words or names e.g., *Neil Diamond – Deil Niamond,* or *John Lennon – Lohn Jennon.* This is a complicated task requiring several operations: segmentation of the initial consonants in both words, transpositions of the initial phonemes, synthesizing new forms. Not only are these cognitive operations demanding but high demands are also made on short-term memory. Younger disordered children could not manage the task, although they were able to identify the initial sounds in monosyllabic words. Twelve- and thirteen-year-old children still had difficulties in managing the task as, e.g., the child who switched initial syllables instead of initial phonemes (*Phil Collins* to *Col Phillins, John Lennon* to *Len Johnen*) (Snowling *et al.,* 1986).

The phoneme-segmentation tasks vary in the degree of difficulty depending on the type of demands they make. In the easiest one the children are asked to say a bit of a word, are asked again until they give a smaller part, and are not required to segment the whole sequence into phonemes but partial segmentation is sufficient, e.g. *boa* as part of *boat.* Higher demands are made in the other two tasks where a complete segmentation of the phonemic sequence is required in order, for instance, to indicate the number of phonemes. In the elision task the child is furthermore required to synthesize the remaining sounds after deleting one segment to yield a new word, a manipulation that cannot be undertaken without awareness of all the elements in the phonemic sequence. In the spoonerism task, it is not sufficient to segment and synthesize, but these operations have to be undertaken on two forms after a transposition of elements which entail high demands on working memory.

Levels of metalinguistic awareness

Reviewing these studies of phonological awareness in language-disordered children, the results on different tasks seem to reflect both the different demands made by the various tasks and different levels or aspects of metalinguistic awareness. From studies where several tasks are given to the same subjects, we can conclude that awareness of syllables seems to develop before awareness of phonemes as linguistic units. That syllables are more easily accessible than linguistic units like phonemes can be explained by the fact that there are direct auditory cues, peaks of acoustic energy, corresponding to the number of syllables. Phonemic segments, on the other hand, are encoded into larger units of syllable size and there is no simple one-to-one correspondence between the phonemic structure and the acoustic speech signal. Thus, phoneme-segmentation tasks are not helped by acoustic information in the continuous speech signal but require an analysis in terms of abstract linguistic units.

Whenever rhyming is included among the tests, these tasks are more easily managed than both syllable and phoneme segmentation. As it is claimed that rhyming requires phonemic awareness, this may seem incompatible with what was said above about the awareness of syllables and phonemes. A possible explanation is that rhyming requires only partial segmentation while a complete segmentation of the phonemic sequence is required in other tasks. Another way of explaining this apparent inconsistency is by adopting the distinction made by Morais *et al.* (1987) between awareness of phonological strings without separate representation of constituents and awareness of phonological units (syllables, phonemes). According to them, rhyming requires the ability to disregard content and to attend to the phonological form. Rhyme may 'depend on sensitivity to phonological similarities without necessarily requiring an analytic competence' (1987: 426), thus reflecting an awareness of phonological strings but no segmental awareness. The same assumption can be made about another of the least problematic metalinguistic tasks, namely to decide whether words are long or short, i.e. a task which requires an awareness of phonological strings but not necessarily of phonemes.

COMPARISONS BETWEEN PHONOLOGICALLY DISORDERED CHILDREN AND NORMAL CHILDREN

In a majority of the reviewed studies comparisons were made between language-disordered children and normally developing children matched to the disordered group on the basis of mental age or language age. In all comparisons, the disordered children managed the tasks less well than the normal children. This was so even if they had the advantage of a more advanced cognitive level, as in comparisons with a control group matched on the basis of language age. Older language-disordered children showed a higher degree of linguistic awareness than younger ones, i.e. their linguistic awareness develops over the years, even if it does not become as advanced as normal children's, and we find examples of individuals in their teens or adults who cannot perform tasks, like rhyming, which normal children manage at an early age.

Comparisons were also made with reading-impaired children with no history of language disorders (Kamhi and Catts, 1986). Contrary to the expectations of the authors, the language-disordered children did not differ significantly from the reading-impaired ones, who even performed slightly more poorly than the language-impaired ones on some tasks (sentence division and phoneme elision). This points in the same direction as the results reported by Magnusson and Nauclér (1987) in a study of language-disordered children and a matched group of normal children. Children who qualified as poor readers, in either the language-disordered group or in the normal one, after the first school year, were children who were metalinguistically unaware, while good readers were children who were metalinguistically aware already at the age of six, one year before they started school. What the poor readers have in common and what differentiates them from the good readers, with or without a history of language disorders, is a low degree of linguistic awareness.

Even if comparisons of language-disordered and normal children at a group level always show disordered children to be less aware than normal children, this pattern is not always observed when comparisons are made at an individual level, as in the Magnusson and Nauclér study (1987). Here normal children had been matched to the disordered ones at an individual level on the basis of age sex and nonverbal cognitive level. When the matched children in the thirty-seven pairs were compared, it was found that in seven pairs the disordered child performed better on all metalinguistic tasks, and in five further pairs the disordered child did better on some, but not all, of the tasks. This pattern was observed at the first testing, when the children were six years old, and remained at all later testings. It is worth mentioning that, at the end of first grade, all of these children were better readers and spellers than their matched normal peers.

INDIVIDUAL VARIATION IN METALINGUISTIC AWARENESS IN PHONOLOGICALLY DISORDERED CHILDREN

Why do phonologically disordered children perform less well than normal children on metalinguistic tasks? Several factors may contribute to the fact that fewer disordered children than normal ones of the same age give evidence of linguistic awareness.

Linguistic awareness varies a lot in normal children and variation in this respect is larger than variation in linguistic production and perception abilities (Tunmer and Herriman, 1984). In language-disordered children the variation in linguistic awareness is even greater. As there are linguistically normal children who are linguistically unaware, it is reasonable to assume that there are disordered children who are unaware for the same reasons: perhaps because their cognitive way of functioning does not allow them to make the product of mental processes an object of thought or, if we adopt Mattingly's definition of linguistic awareness as a person's access to his or her linguistic knowledge, because they have no access to their linguistic knowledge, or they have not had the kind of experiences that are necessary in order to develop an awareness of language. But there are more phonologically unaware children among the disordered children than would be accounted for by this explanation.

Some phonologically disordered children's difficulties in performing metalinguistic tasks may be explained by the kind of linguistic knowledge these children have access to. If their phonological representation is different, they will make incorrect responses on metalinguistic tasks even if they have access to their phonological knowledge just as normal children and have the same ability to analyse. Several observations may be interpreted in this direction.

In the earlier mentioned study of rhyming in twenty-seven phonologically disordered preschool children (Magnusson, 1983), a reanalysis of the children's responses were made. When the children's produced forms differed from the normal forms, the scoring of responses as correct or incorrect was made both in terms of the normal forms and in terms of the produced forms of the particular child. The analysis indicated that children may adopt different strategies: twelve children scored higher if it was assumed that they applied their rhyming strategies, for end rhymes or alliteration, to their own forms instead of to the normal forms. In the first analysis, one child's responses seemed to indicate that he did not understand the task, as he said on several occasions that all the words in the triplets (the two rhyming words and the non-rhyming distractor), or none of them, were rhymes. If it was assumed that his decisions were based on alliterations on his own forms, his responses made sense. On the other hand, some children with very deviant speech got higher scores, if it was assumed that they used normal forms for their rhyming operations.

As was mentioned earlier in the section on rhyming, phonological awareness cannot be predicted from the degree of deviance evidenced in speech production. On the other hand, the type of phonological problems a child have may be critical. Magnusson and Nauclér (1987) made an attempt to relate the observed variance in linguistic awareness to a subclassification of the language-disordered group based on the children's performance on language-production tasks. Children whose phonological problems were predominantly of a segmental nature, manifested as, for instance, substitutions or deletions of phonemes, tended to show a high degree of awareness, while children whose problems were mainly of a sequential nature, manifested as assimilations, metathesis, etc., seemed totally unaware of phonemes, and had vague ideas about syllables. However, they were exceptionally good at judging syntactic acceptability, even if their results on syntactic-production tasks were poor. Children with predominantly syntactic problems, on the other hand, showed a lower degree of linguistic awareness than children with only phonological problems. From this it is evident that children can be aware of linguistic phenomena that they do not use in their own production and that the type of phonological problem is important for the disordered child's performance on metalinguistic tasks, as some types of problems can be assumed to involve a different phonological representation while others do not, at least not in respects that are critical for the completion of tasks designed to measure phonological awareness.

Yet another way that phonologically disordered children's problems may influence their performance on metalinguistic tasks is when discrimination is faulty. As was shown in the section on rhyming, children may demonstrate phonological awareness, in this case an understanding of the rhyming principle, when the test material does not put high demands on auditory discrimination ability, but perform much more poorly when finer auditory discriminations are required. In this case the children could perform the necessary operations, provided that the linguistic material was suited for, and did not exceed, the child's linguistic ability.

Even if a majority of the language-disordered children are less aware than normal children, there are some disordered children who are as, or even more, aware than normal children. How is that possible? A reasonable assumption is that this may be an effect of speech therapy. There are no doubts that linguistic awareness can be trained, at least in normal children (Olofsson and Lundberg, 1983), and this is probably true also for a majority of the disordered children. In the longitudinal study by Magnusson and Nauclér (1987), it was observed that awareness of phonemes increased most rapidly during the first school year, while the children were subject to intensive reading instruction. During the last preschool year, phoneme-segmentation ability did not develop in the disordered group, even if they had speech therapy, while the segmentation ability increased during the same period in normal children who had not been subject to speech therapy, nor to reading instruction. When the group of disordered children who had had speech therapy was compared to a group of disordered children who had not had therapy, the non-therapy group showed more linguistic awareness than the therapy group (Magnusson and Nauclér, 1985). It is reasonable to assume that the therapy children had more serious linguistic problems, but in view of what has been said above about the difficulties of predicting linguistic awareness from the degree of deviance, evidenced in speech production, this does not warrant an assumption of a lower level of linguistic awareness in the therapy group. If, on the other hand, speech therapy were the only critical agent in the development of linguistic awareness in phonologically disordered children, we would expect the therapy group to show a higher level of awareness. Another possibility is that they would have given even less evidence of linguistic awareness, had they not been enrolled in therapy.

The observation by Lagergren and Larsson (1986) also has a bearing on the role of speech therapy for the development of linguistic awareness. They found no differences among their phonologically disordered subjects depending on whether or not they had had speech therapy. The children who had had no therapy had linguistic problems that qualified them for speech therapy, but they were tested before they had been enrolled in the programme.

However, these observations about the role of speech therapy do not exclude the possibility that linguistic awareness can be trained, specifically if programmes are developed with this particular aim. The fact that some phonologically disordered children are more metalinguistically aware than normal children cannot be explained by differences in cognitive capacity, as the children in the Magnusson and Nauclér study had been matched for cognitive level. Nor is the developmental language level more advanced in the phonologically disordered children who show a higher level of metalinguistic awareness than their matched normally developing peers. One possibility is that their linguistic problems are of a type that does not affect their possibilities of becoming linguistically aware. Or the disordered children's better performance is dependent on other factors that have been suggested by Van Kleeck (1984b) to account for the variation in linguistic awareness, e.g. creativity, cognitive style.

With this background, statements like the one by Rack and Snowling (1985: 34) that 'almost by definition, any child who cannot say a word correctly will have difficulty segmenting it at phonemic level' express too simplistic a view of complicated relationships. The fact that a majority of the disordered children managed metalinguistic tasks less well then normal children may be explained in the following way: some children have not developed the cognitive way of functioning that is required in order to reflect upon, analyse, judge or manipulate language and its structural characteristics. They have no access to their linguistic knowledge. Other disordered children may have access to their linguistic knowledge but their knowledge may be more or less deviant. If they use their deviant representations for judgements or manipulations, they may come up with incorrect responses, even if they are as able as normal children to make the required operations and to reflect upon language. If the tasks to assess awareness contain linguistic items for which the representations are not deviant, the same children will give correct responses. For instance, a child may be able to make phonemic segmentations of sequences containing singletons but do not manage the task if sequences contain consonant clusters. If the child considers clusters as one unit instead of two, as in a normal representation, this does not reflect an inability to segment syllables into smaller units but may be the reflection of a different phonological representation. These children are able to reflect upon language but the language that is the object of thought has different structural characteristics. In a third group of disordered children both these circumstances may coincide so that they are not able to reflect upon language and, furthermore, their linguistic knowledge is deviant. Finally, there are language-disordered children who seem to have access to normal phonological representations, even if their speech production is deviant.

Thus both language-disordered and normal children differ in terms of whether or not their knowledge about linguistic structures is accessible and can be made an object of thought. In language-disordered children the situation may further be complicated by the fact that their phonological representations may be different in critical respects. Reasoning along those lines accounts for the facts that more language-disordered than normal children have reading and spelling problems; that poor readers, whether or not they have a history of language disorder, show a lower degree of linguistic awareness than good readers (Kamhi and Catts, 1986; Magnusson and Nauclér 1987); and that some, though not many, language-disordered children develop into good readers and spellers, in spite of their linguistic handicap (Nauclér and Magnusson, forthcoming).

CLINICAL AND EDUCATIONAL IMPLICATIONS

Studies of metalinguistic awareness in phonologically disordered children are consistent in showing a majority of the disordered children to be less aware of language than normal children. The lower degree or lack of linguistic awareness may have far-reaching consequences for the children's development in several ways.

Success in learning to read and write has been shown to be closely related to metalinguistic abilities and, consequently, a majority of language-disordered children have difficulties in acquiring language in its written form. This is apparent not only at the initial stages of literacy but also at later stages, all through the school years and into adulthood, although the problems may take on a different character as the demands made on reading and writing ability change. As a lot of the work at school is dependent on getting information from written texts, it is not surprising that disordered children have academic problems. Both at school and in our highly literate societies at large, heavy demands are made on the ability to read and write. Those children who are linguistically aware, preferably before they start school, stand a much better chance of being successful in spite of their linguistic handicap than children who are linguistically unaware.

The role of linguistic awareness in the development of spoken language is much more unclear. A child who is linguistically aware may use his or her insights in a very conscious way in order to learn more about language, e.g. by asking specific questions about the pronunciation and meaning of words. The systematic variation and practice of structural features that young children engage in as a playful activity when they are on their own, has been suggested as important for developing and gaining control of the phonological system (Ferguson and Macken, 1980). It is difficult to imagine children engaging in such activities without at least some awareness of language form. Do phonologically disordered children discover this pleasurable way of practising and playing with linguistic forms and features?

The language play that older children engage in draws heavily on metalinguistic abilities, e.g. skipping rhymes, ritualized insults, puns, riddles, secret languages. Linguistically unaware children do not understand these kinds of language games and are thereby excluded from a lot of what makes up childhood culture and are not able to take part in these games and activities which serve important social functions in contacts with other children and groups of children. More subtle and creative uses of language, building on structural and lexical ambiguities, or on figurative or metaphorical language, are also beyond the grasp of a majority of the disordered children.

Disordered children who are linguistically aware seem to have a better chance of developing both spoken and written language than children who are linguistically unaware. This is so for children at early developmental levels and, even more so, for children at more advanced linguistic levels. As linguistic awareness seems to be important for several aspects of child development, it must be given due attention in our assessment of phonological disorders and in the planning of intervention programmes.

ASSESSMENT

Even if we are not prepared to accept Van Kleeck's claim (1984b) that all standardized tests are metalinguistic in character as they measure language skills outside a social interactive context, there are some tasks among the test items in currently used language tests that are testing metalinguistic skills, e.g. the sound-blending subtest of the Illinois Test of Psycholinguistic Ability (ITPA) developed by Kirk *et al.* (1968). Psychological tests often include rhymes, synonyms, definitions and anagrams among the subtests for measuring verbal intelligence. On close examination we will find information about metalinguistic skills in the available tests, but in order to assess the level of awareness in a more systematic way, these test items have to be supplemented with other metalinguistic tasks.

In assessing linguistic awareness it may be worthwhile to try to differentiate between children who cannot disregard content and make language and linguistic structures an object of thought from those who can do this but have access to linguistic knowledge that is deviant. Such a differentiation may not be easy to make, but thinking along those lines may be important for the planning of intervention and training. In neither case do the children give the right responses on metalinguistic tasks but in the first case training should, as an initial step, aim at a different attitude towards language, making language opaque (to use Cazden's terminology), instead of just being a means to convey meaning. In the other case, when children are able to reflect upon language, the ability to focus on linguistic form could be used as a means in training with the aim of changing those parts of the child's linguistic system that are deviant. In most children work has to be done in both directions.

From the evaluation of test methods in the review of research, some conclusions can be drawn concerning the requirements on tasks to be used in order to assess linguistic awareness in phonologically disordered children. As many language-disordered children have limited short-term memories, at least for verbal material, the demands on memory should be kept as low as possible. Furthermore, the choice of response mode is important. If possible, a non-verbal response mode is preferable in order to ensure that a child's deviant speech production is not mistaken for lack of linguistic awareness. Tasks which require children to formulate their ideas about language verbally or to give definitions of metalinguistic terms are less appropriate as the disordered children's difficulties in finding linguistic expressions for their ideas may influence their responses negatively. Response modes that put a low demand on verbal formulation and speech production are preferred, e.g. choosing between alternatives, matching, pointing or other non-verbal response modes. Attention should also be given to the difficulty of the various tasks, ensuring that a child will not be considered, for instance, unaware of phonemes after being tested with a difficult task like elision of phonemes without trying more easily managed tasks, e.g. phoneme identification. The choice of linguistic material used in the tasks should also be considered as the performance of children on their way of becoming linguistically aware may be influenced by the phonetic substance of the test items.

INTERVENTION

An important issue in relation to intervention is whether or not metalinguistic awareness can be trained. Several studies, e.g. Olofsson and Lundberg (1983) and Morais (1985), show that normal children become more aware of language, and improve their reading and spelling, after training on tasks involving metalinguistic skills. However, some children did not seem to profit from the training. No systematic training studies have been done on phonologically disordered children, but some information about the role of training can be gained from longitudinal study of disordered children enrolled in therapy as preschoolers and subject to phonic training as part of reading instruction at school (Magnusson and Nauclér, 1987). During the time the children had reading instruction, their awareness of phonemes increased most rapidly. This is also so for those children who do not learn to read. During the time the children had speech therapy the increase in phoneme awareness was not equally obvious but, on the other hand, the intervention programmes used did not specifically aim at the development of linguistic awareness.

Although there is some controversy about whether or not to consider children's repairs of their own utterances as evidence for linguistic awareness, there are no doubts that an awareness of communicative failure or requests for clarification from the listener make children repair their utterances and may lead them to consider and, eventually, to discover the linguistic structure of the utterance as a possible source of the communicative failure. If they are able to analyse structural features, they may try to change structural characteristics in attempts to get their meaning across.

Spontaneous repairs have not been studied in language-disordered children but there is some information about how they respond to requests for clarifications. Gallagher and Darnton (1978) compared twelve language-disordered children's revision behaviours to that of normal children at the same linguistic level, Brown's stages I, II, and III. The subjects had 'no clinically significant articulatory deviations' and had been subject to therapy between six months and three years. When they were not understood, the children responded by revising the previous utterance (75 per cent) or repeating it (17 per cent). 8 per cent did not respond when asked to clarify utterances that were not understood. Revision strategies were the same, independent of language stage, and were not determined by the structural knowledge at each stage as for the normal children. At all stages the disordered children changed the phonetic shape (31 per cent), reduced (33 per cent), elaborated (29 per cent) or substituted (7 per cent) constituents which seemed to be chosen at random. Each disordered child had his or her own selection of revision strategies that were used in an unsystematic and undifferentiated way relative to his or her structural knowledge or the structural characteristics of the utterance.

Brinton *et al.* (1986) investigated disordered children's responses to stacked sequences of requests for clarification in order to study how language-disordered children adapt to the listener in a situation where the listener does not understand the message in spite of the speaker's repeated attempts to repair. Thirty disordered children in the ages 4;10 to 9;10 were compared to thirty normal children in the same ages. Severe 'speech articulation problems' were excluded but especially in the youngest group, children made some sound substitutions. At the first request, 87 per cent tried to repair but for each request in the sequence the number of repairs decreased, especially for the language-disordered children, who did not persist in repeating the utterance or who could not think of anything else to try. Repetition was the most frequent repair in all groups but for each request in the sequence, the number of repetitions decreased as the younger and the disordered children made more inappropriate responses and the older and the normal children added information or gave cues to the context or the background. Few of the children changed the form of the utterance but some revised the phonetic forms without making phoneme substitutions, e.g. by lengthening vowels or aspirating final stops.

That language-impaired children, like young normal children, are apt to blame the listener for communicative failures in judgements of inadequate messages has been shown by Meline and Brackin (1987). Language-disordered children have difficulties in realizing that messages that are too general are inadequate not because of the listener but because of the speaker's non-specific requests.

What we can conclude from these studies of language-disordered children's repairs and judgements of communicative failures is that they do not use repair strategies in the same way as normal children do and that they have difficulties in realizing why messages fail, although they seem to recognize the necessity to repair their previous utterance when the listener requires clarification. They seem to blame the listener for the communicative failure and have problems in revising the form of their utterances in a way that is appropriate in a given situation.

That language-disordered children have difficulties in changing the structural form of utterances even if they are aware that the structural form is not correct has been shown in studies of children's judgement and subsequent corrections of unacceptable sentences. Magnusson and Nauclér (1987), in a longitudinal study of language-disordered children in the ages six to eight years, had the children judge the syntactic/morphological acceptability of sentences and to correct those sentences that they had found unacceptable. Even children who showed their metalinguistic awareness by being correct in their judgement of forms, had considerable difficulties in correcting ungrammatical structures.

With this background it is evident that phonologically disordered children need help to realize why their utterances are not understood, to focus on the linguistic structure of the utterance and to learn how to change linguistic forms and features. Dean and Howell (1986) have outlined an intervention programme based on similar ideas, where they make explicit use of children's awareness of communicative failure and of structural features of the phonological system as an intervention strategy with phonologically disordered children. Work is directed at developing the children's awareness of the sound system and of communicative effectiveness. No work is done on speech-sound production but is directed at changing the underlying rule system, thereby changing the output. In the first phase of therapy, work is directed at developing the child's awareness of structural aspects of language and the ability to reflect upon and manipulate them, which is a prerequisite for a more effective use of repairs. In the second phase work is directed at communicative effectiveness by giving feedback about the child's success or failure to convey meaning, without drawing direct attention to pronunciation. By this procedure the child is induced to review his or her utterance, to reflect upon it, and to utilize this increased knowledge of the sound structure to repair his or her utterance which, in the long run, will cause a change in the processing of his or her sound system.

Contrary to intervention programmes, which are more or less based on the implicit assumption that phonologically disordered children are linguistically aware (which a majority of them are not), programmes of the type described above not only make a systematic and conscious use of awareness to promote the development of disordered language but specifically direct work at developing children's awareness of the phonological system and of its use in communication. Therapy based on such considerations may be profitable both for the normalization of spoken language and for the acquisition of reading and writing. As we have seen earlier, disordered children who are linguistically aware learn to read and write without too much trouble while linguistically unaware children have considerable problems, probably both as a consequence of being linguistically unaware and as a result of their deviant language. Whether or not all phonologically disordered children will profit from intervention aiming at developing and using awareness as a therapeutic tool is an empirical question.

REFERENCES

Bertelson, P. (1986) 'The onset of literacy, *Cognition* 24: 1–30.

Bradley, L. and Bryant, P. (1985) *Rhyme and Reason in Reading and Spelling* (International Academy for Research in Learning Disabilities, Monograph Series, 1), Ann Arbor: The University of Michigan Press.

Brinton, B., Fujiki, M., Winkler, E. and Loeb, D.F. (1986) 'Responses to requests for clarification in linguistically normal and language-impaired children', *Journal of Speech and Hearing Disorders* 51: 370–7.

Bruce, D.J. (1964) 'The analysis of word sounds by young children', *British Journal of Educational Psychology* 34: 158–70.

Calfee, R.C. and associates (1980) 'Stanford Foundation Skills Test', book B: 'Phonetic segmentation', unpublished, Stanford University.

Cazden, C.B. (1976) 'Play with language and metalinguistic awareness: one dimension of language experience', in J.S. Bruner, A. Jolly and K. Sylva (eds) *Play*, New York: Basic Books, 603–18.

Clark, E. (1978) 'Awareness of language: some evidence from what children say and do', in A. Sinclair, R. Jarvella and W. Levelt (eds) *The Child's Conception of Language*, Berlin: Springer, 17–44.

Curtiss, S. (1977) *Genie. A Psycholinguistic Study of a Modernday 'Wild Child'*, New York: Academic Press.

Dean, E. and Howell J. (1986) 'Developing linguistic awareness: a theoretically based approach to phonological disorders', *British Journal of Disorders of Communication* 21: 223–38.

Dodd, B. and Hermelin, B. (1977) 'Phonological coding by the prelinguistically deaf', *Perception and Psychophysics* 21: 413–17.

Ehri, L.C. (1984) 'How orthography alters spoken language competences in children learning to read and spell', in J. Downing and R. Valtin (eds) *Language awareness and learning to read*, Berlin: Springer, 119–48.

Ferguson, C.A. and Macken, M.A. (1980) 'Phonological development in children: play and cognition', *Papers and Reports on Child Language Development* 18: 138–77.

Fox, B. and Routh, D. (1975) 'Analyzing spoken language into words, syllables, and phonemes: a developmental study', *Journal of Psycholinguistic Research* 4: 331–42.

Fudge, E.C. (1969) 'Syllables', *Journal of Linguistics* 5: 253–86.

Gallagher, T. and Darnton, B. (1978) 'Conversational aspects of the speech of language-disordered children: revision behaviors', *Journal of Speech and Hearing Research* 21: 118–35.

Hakes, D. (1980) *The Development of Metalinguistic Abilities in Children*, Berlin: Springer.

Hirsh-Pasek, K., Gleitman, L. and Gleitman, H. (1978) 'What did the brain say to the mind? A study of the detection and report of ambiguity by young children', in A. Sinclair, R. Jarvella and W. Levelt (eds) *The Child's Conception of Language*, Berlin: Springer, 97–132.

Kamhi, A.G. and Catts, H.W. (1986) 'Toward an understanding of developmental language and reading disorders', *Journal of Speech and Hearing Disorders* 51: 337–47.

Kamhi, A.G., Lee, R. and Nelson, L. (1985) 'Word, syllable, and sound awareness in language-disordered children', *Journal of Speech and Hearing Disorders* 50: 207–13.

Kirk, S., McCarthy, J. and Kirk, W. (1968) *The Illinois Test of Psycholinguistic Abilities*, Urbana: The University of Illinois Press.

Lagergren, C. and Larsson, A. (1986) 'Språklig medvetenhet hos tal- och språkförsenade barn' (Linguistic awareness in speech- and language-delayed children), Examensarbete i logopedi, Institutionen för logopedi och foniatri, Karolinska institutet, Huddinge sjukhus (Final term paper in logopaedics, Karolinska institute, Huddinge hospital).

Liberman, I.Y., Shankweiler, C., Liberman, A.M., Fowler, C. and Fischer, F.W. (1977) 'Phonetic segmentation and recoding in the beginning reader', in A.S. Reber and D.L. Scarborough (eds) *Towards a Psychology of Reading*, Proceedings of the CUNY conference, Hillsdale, NJ: Lawrence Erlbaum Associates, 207–25

Magnusson, E. (1983) *The Phonology of Language Disordered Children: Production, Perception, and Awareness* (Travaux de l'Institut de linguistique de Lund, XVII), Lund: Gleerups.

Magnusson, E. and Nauclér, K. (1985) 'Linguistic awareness, cognitive level, and short term memory in language disordered and normally speaking pre-school children', paper presented at the first International Congress of Applied Psycholinguistics, 16–20 June, Barcelona.

Magnusson, E. and Nauclér, K. (1987) 'Language disordered and normally speaking children's development of spoken and written language: preliminary results from a longitudinal study', *RUUL, Reports from Uppsala University*, Department of Linguistics 16: 36–63.
Magnusson, E., Nauclér, K. and Söderpalm, E. (1984) 'Form or substance? The linguistic awareness of pre-school children and school children investigated by means of rhyming test', *Working Papers*, Department of Linguistics, Lund University 27: 165–78.
Marshall, J.C. and Morton, J. (1978) 'On the mechanics of EMMA', in A. Sinclair, R.J. Jarvella and W.J.M. Levelt (eds) *The Child's Conception of Language*, Berlin: Springer, 225–40.
Mattingly, I. (1972) 'Reading, the linguistic process, and linguistic awareness', in J. Kavanagh and I. Mattingly (eds) *Language by Ear and by Eye: the Relationships between Speech and Reading*, Cambridge, MA: MIT Press, 133–48.
Meline, T.J. and Bracklin, S.R. (1987) 'Language-impaired children's awareness of inadequate messages', *Journal of Speech and Hearing Disorders* 52: 263–70.
Morais, J. (1985) 'Phonetic awareness and reading acquisition', paper presented to the inaugural meeting of the European Society for Cognitive Psychology, Nijmegen, 9–12 September.
Morais, J., Alegria, J. and Content A. (1987) 'The relationships between segmental analysis and alphabetic literacy: an interactive view', *Cahiers de Psychologie Cognitive, European Bulletin of Cognitive Psychology* 7: 415–38.
Nauclér, K. and Magnusson, E. (1985) 'Language disordered children's reading and spelling: preliminary results', *Working Papers*, Department of Linguistics, Lund University 28: 127–37.
Nauclér, K. and Magnusson, E. (forthcoming) 'How to become a good reader and speller in spite of linguistic disabilities', In *Praktisk Lingvistik*, Department of Linguistics, Lund University.
Nesdale, A.R., Herriman, M.L. and Tunmer, W.E. (1984) 'Phonological awareness in children', in W.E. Tunmer, J.C. Pratt and M.L. Herriman (eds) *Metalinguistic Awareness in Children*. Berlin: Springer, 56–72.
Olofsson, A. and Lundberg, I. (1983) 'Can phonemic awareness be trained in kindergarten?' *Scandinavian Journal of Psychology* 24: 35–44.
Papandropoulou, I. and Sinclair, H. (1974) 'What is a word? Experimental study of children's ideas on grammar', *Human Development* 17: 241–58.
Perin, D. (1983) 'Phoneme segmentation and spelling', *British Journal of Psychology* 74: 129–45.
Pratt, C. and Nesdale, A.R. (1984) 'Pragmatic awareness in children', in W.E. Tunmer, J.C. Pratt and M.L. Herriman (eds) *Metalinguistic Awareness in Children*, Berlin: Springer, 105–25.
Rack, J. and Snowling, M. (1985) 'Verbal deficits in dyslexia: a review', in M.J. Snowling (ed.) *Children's Written Language Difficulties*, Windsor: NFER-Nelson, 28–42.
Sinclair, H. (1978) 'Conceptualization and awareness in Piaget's theory and

its relevance to the child's conception of language', in A. Sinclair, R.J. Jarvella and W.J.M. Levelt (eds) *The Child's Conception of Language*, Berlin: Springer, 191–200.

Snowling, M.J., Stackhouse, J., and Rack, J. (1986) 'Phonological dyslexia and dysgraphia – a developmental study', *Cognitive Neuropsychology* 3: 309–99.

Stackhouse, J. (1985) 'Segmentation, speech and spelling difficulties', in M.J. Snowling (ed.) *Children's Written Language Difficulties*, Windsor: NFER-Nelson, 96–115.

Stackhouse, J. and Snowling, M. (1983) 'Segmentation and spelling in children with speech disorders', paper presented at XIX congress of the International Association of Logopaedics and Phoniatrics, Edinburgh, 14–18 August.

Treiman, R. (1983) 'The structure of spoken syllables: evidence from novel word games', *Cognition* 15: 49–74.

Tunmer, W.E. and Herriman, M.L. (1984) 'The development of meta-linguistic awareness: a conceptual view', in W.E. Tunmer, J.C. Pratt and M.L. Herriman (eds) *Metalinguistic Awareness in Children*, Berlin: Springer 12–35.

Valtin, R. (1984) 'Awareness of features and functions of language', in J. Downing and R. Valtin (eds) *Language Awareness and Learning to Read*, Berlin: Springer, 227–60.

Van Kleeck, A. (1984a) 'Metalinguistic skills: cutting across spoken and written language and problem solving abilities', in G.P. Wallach and K. Butler (eds) *Language Learning Disabilities in School Age Children*, Baltimore: Williams & Wilkins, 128–53.

Van Kleeck A. (1984b) 'Assessment and intervention: does "meta" matter?' in G.P. Wallach and K. Butler (eds) *Language Learning Disabilities in School Age Children*, Baltimore: Williams & Wilkins, 179–98.

Weir R. (1962) *Language in the Crib*, The Hague: Mouton.

Vygotsky L.S. (1962) *Thought and Language*, Cambridge, MA: MIT Press.

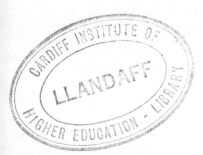

5   Functional considerations in phonological assessment of child speech

Eeva Leinonen

Phonological disability in children is characterized by loss of contrasts in the phonological system, thus potentially restricting the ability of that system to signal meaning differences in language. Such systems are said to be communicatively (Grunwell, 1985) or functionally (Leinonen, 1988) inadequate. The aim of phonological assessment is to identify the absence of which contrasts contributes to the communicative or functional inadequacy of the system and to prioritize these in terms of their detrimental effect on the signalling of meaning differences (Leinonen, 1988). This in turn feeds into the planning of remedial goals, aiming to improve the communicative and functional adequacy of the phonological system. The purpose of this chapter is to explore the notions of communicative and functional (in)adequacy of children's phonological systems and to comment on the implications of this exploration for the assessment and management of phonological disorders in children. Specific attention is paid to homophony as an index of functional inadequacy.

COMMUNICATIVE AND FUNCTIONAL (IN)ADEQUACY

The term 'communicative adequacy' can be interpreted differently depending on whether one takes a narrow or a broad view of the term 'communicative'. Taking a narrow view (Grunwell, 1985), a phonological system is communicatively inadequate if contrasts required to signal meaning differences in the ambient language are missing. As such, communicative inadequacy reflects the differences in contrastive phones in the child and adult (target) phonological systems and the extent of potential homophony in the child's lexical system which the phonological system serves to support. To widen this view slightly, it can be assumed that homophony in children's lexical systems is reflected in their spoken language, which in turn may hinder the recoverability of meanings by listeners. When interpreting communicative adequacy in the narrow sense, the focus is on the child's system rather than on the consequences this system may have for the sharing of meanings in communicative contexts.

Contrasting with this narrow view, we can interpret 'communicative adequacy' to reflect the real consequences restricted phonological systems can have on sharing of meanings. In doing so, we need to consider what listeners find difficult to interpret and how this relates to the child's phonological system, to the ability of listeners to interpret meanings and to the communicative situation. Focusing on the child, we need to ask what it is in his or her phonological system which can hinder the interpretation of meanings by the listener. Following Connolly (1984) and others (e.g. Grunwell, 1985; Leinonen, 1988) homophony and variability in child realizations may hinder recoverability of meanings, as can the auditory distance of the adult target sound (word) and its child realization (Line, 1987) and the frequency of the abnormality. The child's phonological problem may also interact with other language, or cognitive, motor or other such problems to render his or her utterances uninterpretable. Focusing on the listener, ambiguous or unclear messages reflecting disordered phonological systems may or may not become processed depending on the listener's ability to interpret meanings (e.g. native vs foreign speakers) or his or her familiarity with the child. Contextual and co-textual cues may also hinder or aid interpretation. The child's utterances reflecting a disordered phonological system may become clarified by, for instance, accompanying non-verbal behaviour. Thus, when taking a broad view of what constitutes a communicatively (in)adequate phonological system we venture beyond strictly linguistic considerations to the domains of human cognition and pragmatics.

As researchers, we can take a narrow view of communicative adequacy and study phonological disability in such decontextualized terms. But can speech-language clinicians do so when their aim is to help the child to become a communicator? There is no simple answer to this. On the one hand, clinicians do increasingly appreciate the wider contextual influences which shape communicative encounters and can thus affect one's view of communicative ability or disability (Smith and Leinonen, forthcoming). However, because of lack of analytical, intergrative frameworks for analysing and interpreting clients' language disability within wider contexts, one necessarily concentrates on smaller components. Furthermore, despite being able to communicate, be it by contextual help or because of the listener's powers of interpretation, the child needs a system of phonological contrasts in order to have a chance of functioning as a communicator beyond familiar communicative contexts. Yet, by concentrating on the phonological system in one's clinical approach, caution needs to be exercised not to dismiss the importance of interaction of factors which may render a phonological system communicatively adequate or inadequate. That is to say that absence of phonological contrasts from the system may not have communicative consequences.

Current approaches to phonological disability take a narrow view of phonological systems and their adequacy. This can be extended without attempting to incorporate the broadest view into practice. A workable approach begins with modest goals, based on the analysis of separate factors which potentially contribute towards communicative inadequacy of a phonological system. The outcome of such an analysis can then be incorporated into assessment procedures, enabling one to speculate on the potential communicative consequences of restricted phonological systems in a systematic and principled way. Leinonen (1987, 1988) devised a means of assessing the extent of potential homophony in children's lexical systems resulting from lack of contrasts in phonological systems. While this essentially refers to the narrow view of communicative inadequacy, in order to avoid making the distinction between the narrow and broad views, the term 'functional (in)adequacy' is used instead. The assessment of the functional adequacy of children's phonological systems has direct implications for the planning of remedial goals, aiming to reduce systematically potential homophony in children's lexical systems and their speech.

Homophony reduction can be considered a well-motivated goal in the clinical management of phonological disability. The function of the phonological system is lexical differentiation, and thus assessment and remediation based on the principle of maximally restoring the functioning of the phonological system is an obvious goal in treatment. This is a reasonable goal even if we can only deal with meaning differentiation in lexical systems rather than in communication. This, together with the potential detrimental effect of homophony on the recoverability of meaning differences by listeners, promotes the establishment of missing contrasts into children's phonological systems on this basis. It is also more realistic to target potential homophony rather than attempt to assess and reduce actual homophony (see Ingram, 1981; Grunwell, 1985) given the generally limited data samples upon which phonological analyses in clinical contexts are based.

ASSESSING FUNCTIONAL (IN)ADEQUACY

The concept and measure of functional loss (FLOSS) has been developed (Leinonen, 1987, 1988) to gauge the extent of homophony in lexical systems reflecting the loss of contrasts in the phonological system. This measure, together with a means of predicting potential homophony in lexical systems, enables one to assess the functional (in)adequacy of phonological systems. In this section, the measure of FLOSS will be first outlined, then methods for predicting potential homophony without recourse to ready calculated FLOSS values will be discussed and finally a study in which FLOSS values were calculated is briefly discussed (Leinonen, 1987, 1988). Implications of these explorations for the assessment and remediation of phonological disorders in children are then considered in the following two sections.

If we assume a lexical system or inventory which consists of lexical entries, the phonological system which serves to support the lexical system provides the only means of differentiating between these entries in terms of their form. Measuring FLOSS in the phonological system on such a basis can be referred to as the assessment of the functional adequacy of the phonological system. In measuring FLOSS the term 'functional' is interpreted in the narrowest of senses: that is, the function of the phonological system is lexical differentiation *per se*. No note is taken of the possibility of homophones occurring in similar or different contexts, of the frequency of occurrence of homophones and other such contextual factors (but see below). Work is currently in progress to address contextual influences bearing upon FLOSS.

FLOSS is measured in terms of the number of *homophonous pairs* in a lexical system resulting from the loss (absence) of contrasts in the phonological system. A homophonous pair consists of two homophonous types which share the same homophonous form (Ingram, 1975). Homophonous types can also be referred to as the lexical targets and homophonous forms as the lexical realizations, e.g.:

$$\left. \begin{array}{c} /\text{spɒt}/ \\ \\ /\text{pɒt}/ \end{array} \right\} \longrightarrow /\text{pɒt}/$$

/spɒt/ and /pɒt/ form a homophonous pair, since they are two homophonous types (i.e. different lexical targets) which share the same homophonous form (i.e. a lexical realization /pɒt/). The homophonous pair indicates a lexical (meaning) distinction which is unsignalled owing to the loss of the contrast /sp–p/ in the word-initial position.

More than one phonological contrast is likely to be missing from a child's phonological system at any one time. The missing contrasts may or may not *conspire* to the same sound segment. Conspiring contrasts are those which have the same phonemic realization for different target sounds (e.g. /s–t/ /k–t/ and /d–t/). When contrasts conspire they have potential for producing *multiple homophony* and when they do not conspire they do not have this potential. Multiple homophony occurs when more than two homophonous types share the same homophonous form, e.g.:

$$\left. \begin{array}{l} /\text{spɪt}/ \\ /\text{pɪt}/ \\ /\text{bɪt}/ \end{array} \right\} \longrightarrow /\text{pɪt}/$$

Because of the conspiracy of the missing contrasts /sp–p/ and /b–p/ in the word-initial place in structure and the resultant multiple homophony, the number of lexical distinctions left unsignalled is three (i.e. FLOSS = 3). That is to say that the number of homophonous pairs is three (i.e. /spɪt/ vs /pɪt/; /spɪt/ vs /bɪt/; /pɪt/ vs /bɪt/). A linear increase in the number of homophonous types sharing the same homophonous form is (potentially) reflected in a non-linear increase in the FLOSS. Thus, when four homophonous types share the same homophonous form the FLOSS is potentially six, for five types to one form the FLOSS is potentially ten and so on. This relationship of the homophonous types to forms and the FLOSS (i.e. homophonous pairs) can be captured in the following equation (see Connolly, 1980):

$$\frac{N(N-1)}{2}$$

where N signifies the number of homophonous types sharing the same homophonous form.

To reflect the current predominance of phonological process analysis as a descriptive tool in phonological assessment (e.g. Weiner, 1979; Shriberg and Kwiatkowski, 1980; Ingram, 1981; Grunwell, 1985) FLOSS will be discussed in terms of phonological processes herewith. This provides some additional guidelines for functional assessment by introducing the possibility of interaction (or ordering) of processes (see below). The absence of the contrasts /st–t/, /t–d/ and /k–t/ from a phonological system can be described as cluster-reduction, voicing and fronting processes (Stampe, 1979) respectively. Differing from the common practice in phonological process analysis, it is, however, necessary to refer to each subprocess reflecting a loss of contrast as a phonological process and the processes reflecting a group of subprocesses as a process category. Thus, the process category 'fronting' consists of the processes /k–t/, /g–d/ and /ŋ–n/. Furthermore, process analysis is suitable for the present purposes since it captures the unidirectional nature of lost contrasts in children's systems by specifying what the target and its realization tend to be. For instance, if we specify the process /k–t/, or contrast /k–t/, this indicates that the target /k/ is realized by /t/ but not that the target /t/ is realized by /k/.

PREDICTING POTENTIAL FLOSS

By observing the nature of phonological processes and process combinations operative in children's speech, it is possible to make certain predictions about the potential homophony in a child's lexical system resulting from the absence of contrasts in the phonological system. Being able to make such predictions provides a more flexible clinical approach to assessment and remediation (see below). One is not dependent on ready-calculated FLOSS values for all the processes present in any one child's speech but is offered more general guidelines for exploring the functional consequences of restricted phonological systems.

As indicated above, if one phonological contrast is missing from the phonological system (i.e. only one process operates) no multiple homophony can be produced in the lexical system. This is also the case if more than one contrast is missing but none of the contrasts conspire to the same sound segment. In both instances, homophony can only be produced by homophonous forms matching with lexical items present in the lexical system, and which are part of the lexicon of the ambient language. With regard to conspiring contrasts (processes) this does not necessarily need to be so. Compare (a) and (b) below:

(a)   /tr–t/, /dr–t/ and /d–t/ conspiring

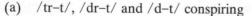

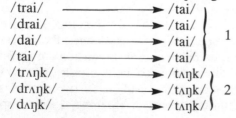

(1) signifies homophonous forms which are part of the ambient language and (2) those which are not.

(b) /tr–t/ and /g–d/ non-conspiring

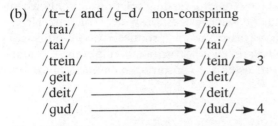

(3) and (4) signify homophonous forms which are not part of the ambient language.

This example illustrates how conspiring contrasts or processes can produce homophony both via matching lexical items in the ambient language and lexical forms not part of the ambient language, while non-conspiring processes can only produce homophony via the former. This difference, reflecting a difference in potential for multiple homophony, renders conspiring processes potentially more detrimental for the functional adequacy of the phonological system than non-conspiring processes. This enables one to predict potential homophony without recourse to ready-calculated FLOSS values.

Thus, assessing the functional adequacy of children's phonological systems involves determining which contrasts or processes are non-conspiring and which are conspiring. When operating within a phonological process framework it is essential to recognize that apparently non-conspiring processes may end up conspiring if they enter a process relationship (if the processes interact). Only feeding and counter-feeding relationships are considered here, but see further Leinonen (1987). Also, for the sake of clarity we shall consider only combinations of two processes here. The processes /tr–t/ and /t–d/ operating in the word-initial position can be said to be conspiring via entering a feeding relationship if the output of the first process provides input for the second process (Kiparsky, 1968).

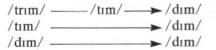

The cluster-reduction process feeds into the voicing process, thus rendering the contrasts /tr–d/ and /t–d/ missing from the phonological system. In this way, the apparently non-conspiring processes have potential for multiple homophony and thus are potentially more detrimental for the functional adequacy of the phonological system than non-conspiring processes proper (single processes) which do not interact via feeding.

Processes can conspire and enter a feeding relationship only when the processes operate in the same place in a word structure. However, multiple homophony can also be produced when processes operate on different places in word structure in different or same words. Whether these processes are conspiring or non-conspiring is incidental.

(a) Different Words
     Process 1: l–w (SIWI)
     Process 2: k–t (SFWF)
     /leit/ ———————➤ /weit/
     /weik/ ———————➤ /weit/
     /weit/ ———————➤ /weit/

(b) Same Words
     Process 1: l–w (SIWI)
     Process 2: k–t (SFWF)
     /leik/ ——— /weik/———➤ /weit/
     /weit/ ————————➤ /weit/

(SIWI = syllable-initial, word-initial; SFWF = syllable-final, word-final.)

As is apparent, (a) has potential for multiple homophony while (b) has not. To keep this discussion to manageable proportions we shall not pursue these types of process operations further but shall concentrate on processes operating in the same place in word structure. For further information on processes operating in different places in word structure, see Leinonen (1987).

When contrasts or processes are non-conspiring and totally non-interacting and when only one process operates at a time on a word, FLOSS simply equals the sum of the FLOSS values for the respective single processes (i.e. when only one contrast is missing from the phonological system). Non-conspiring processes can, however, interact via counter-feeding (Newton, 1971; also displaced contrast, Kiparsky and Menn, 1977) which provides an exception to this principle of additive FLOSS values. A counter-feeding relationship is an opposite to a feeding relationship. When two processes enter a counter-feeding relationship, the homophony produced equals the homophony produced by the process which is ordered first in the counter-feeding relationship. That is to say that the potential for homophony by the second process is lost.

/t–d/ and /k–t/ in a counter-feeding relationship (SIWI)

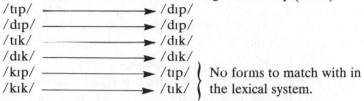

/tɪp/ ⟶ /dɪp/
/dɪp/ ⟶ /dɪp/
/tɪk/ ⟶ /dɪk/
/dɪk/ ⟶ /dɪk/
/kɪp/ ⟶ /tɪp/ ⎫ No forms to match with in
/kɪk/ ⟶ /tɪk/ ⎭ the lexical system.

The fronting process (/k–t/) cannot produce any homophony since all the forms in the lexical system with which the resultant forms could have matched have undergone the prevocalic voicing process (t–d), thus preventing any potential homophony.

There is one further observation which can be made in relation to processes and FLOSS. FLOSS is a reflection of the loss of contrasts. There are, however, processes which as single processes do not conflate contrasts (e.g. glottal replacement in relation to the Received Pronunciation in British English). As such, there is no potential for FLOSS when they operate as single processes. In addition, they can enter into conspiring relationships only within their own process categories or into a feeding relationship as the fed process.

Conspiring	Feeding
Process 1: k–ʔ	Process 1: k–t
Process 2: t–ʔ	↓
	Process 2: t–ʔ

/sæk/ ⟶ /sæʔ/   /sæk/——/sæt/⟶/sæʔ/
/sæt/ ⟶ /sæʔ/   /sæt/ ⟶ /sæʔ/

When either conspiring or entering a feeding relationship, no multiple homophony can be produced by combinations of two such processes. This is because only one phonological contrast is lost (e.g. /k–t/ in SFWF position in the above examples). These types of processes which do not conflate contrasts as single processes also differ from the conflating type in that counter-feeding relationships consisting such processes have no potential for FLOSS. The ability to produce homophony by the second process is still lost, with the difference that the first process cannot produce any homophony either, e.g.:

Process 1: t–ʔ
Process 2: k–t

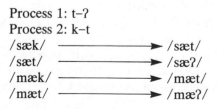

/sæk/ ⟶ /sæt/
/sæt/ ⟶ /sæʔ/
/mæk/ ⟶ /mæt/
/mæt/ ⟶ /mæʔ/

By examining the potential of processes and process relationships for homophony, it is possible to make predictions about FLOSS in the phonological system. We can distinguish three broad categories which reflect potential increase in FLOSS:

1 Processes that have no potential for homophony:
   (a) processes which do not conflate phonological contrasts and which operate as single processes (e.g. glottal replacement and other such processes with a sound realization not part of the phonological system of the ambient language);
   (b) such non-conflicting processes when entering a counter-feeding relationship.
2 Processes that have no potential for multiple homophony:
   (a) non-conspiring processes (i.e. processes not interacting with other processes);
   (b) counter-feeding processes;
   (c) conspiring and feeding processes involving non-conflating processes.
3 Processes that have potential for multiple homophony:
   (a) conspiring processes;
   (b) feeding processes.

Categories 1–3 reflect increasing potential for FLOSS in the phonological system as a function of the nature of phonological processes and combinations of processes found in children's speech.

Categories 2 and 3 can be explored further in terms of their *compatibility or incompatibility with new homophony*. Process combinations which are incompatible with new homophony do not have the potential for producing new instances of homophony as compared to the homophony produced if the processes operated as single processes. All the types of process relationships in (2) (excepting those described in (c)) are incompatible with new homophony. The consequence of this is that FLOSS can be measured in terms of the FLOSS values for the single processes. More specifically:

1 For non-conspiring processes the FLOSS is simply the sum of the FLOSS values for all the respective single processes (in effect, non-conspiring processes are single processes).
2 For counter-feeding processes the FLOSS equals the FLOSS for the first process when operating as a single process.
3 For conspiring and feeding processes involving non-conflating processes the situation is rather different. There are no FLOSS values for single processes since as single processes these processes

have no potential for homophony. Thus, these process relationships cannot be described in terms of (in)compatibility with new homophony.

Those process combinations which have potential for producing multiple homophony (i.e. 3 above) are potentially compatible with new homophony. That is to say that new instances of homophony can be produced as a function of the processes entering a combination. That is also to say that, potentially, the FLOSS is greater than the FLOSS for the respective single processes (but see below). Considering the potential (in)compatibility of processes with new homophony provides a means of estimating potential functional consequences of phonological processes without the need to have ready-calculated FLOSS values for all the processes and process combinations.

The broad categories of 2 and 3 will be further refined after discussing results of a study which calculated FLOSS values for processes. The potential implications and applications for the assessment and management of phonological disorders in children will then be considered.

CALCULATION OF FLOSS VALUES

While certain predictions can be made about the potential functional consequences of children's restricted phonological systems, these predictions can be refined by considering a study in which FLOSS values were calculated. These values are also relevant for future work and study (see below). FLOSS values for phonological processes most commonly found to be operating in the speech of phonologically normal and disordered children have been calculated on the basis of a lexical sample reflecting children's 'common' vocabulary (see Leinonen, 1987, 1988). These were obtained for each process separately and for certain combinations of two processes (see below). The details of the study will not be outlined here; the reader is directed to the above references for further information. Some of the main features and findings, however, need to be reiterated for later discussion.

FLOSS values were calculated for phonological processes commonly found in the speech of phonologically normal and disordered children (Appendix A) when one process at a time operated on the data sample and in combinations of two. We shall consider only those process combinations here which operated in the same place in word structure and were potentially compatible with new homophony (see 3 above). The FLOSS were measured in relation to a lexical sample of 1,836 non-inflected lexical entries which reflect children's (aged 5:11–6:11) 'common' vocabulary as outlined by Burrough (1957). In the calculations, no note was taken of the fact that processes may apply on only certain lexical items or only in certain contexts. FLOSS for each single process was calculated in the syllable-initial word-initial, syllable-final within word (SFWW), syllable-initial within word (SIWW) and syllable-final word-final positions and for the combinations of processes in the SIWI and SFWF positions only.

Rather expectedly, it was found that when one process at a time operated (i.e. one contrast at a time was missing from the system), not much homophony resulted in the lexical system. The mean FLOSS values for the single processes were $\bar{x} = 4.67$ (SD = 4.85) in the SIWI position and $\bar{x} = 7.43$ (SD = 9.53) in the SFWF. Processes operative in the within-word positions had a very marginal effect on FLOSS. No instances of homophony were produced in the SFWW position and the mean FLOSS for the SIWW was $\bar{x} = 0.22$ (SD = 0.66).

Mean FLOSS values for the different process categories (see above) were also calculated in the SIWI and SFWF positions. The following rank order can be established on the basis of these values:

SIWI
1 Fronting ($\bar{x} = 11.50$; SD = 12.03)
2 Gliding ($\bar{x} = 7.00$; SD = 5.60)
3 Prevocalic voicing ($\bar{x} = 6.00$; SD = 7.85)
4 Stopping ($\bar{x} = 5.10$; SD = 4.23)
5 WI cluster reduction ($\bar{x} = 3.27$; SD = 2.68)

SFWF
1 Final-consonant deletion ($\bar{x} = 11.00$; SD = 11.44)
2 Fronting ($\bar{x} = 7.00$; SD = 11.55)
3 WF devoicing ($\bar{x} = 5.00$; SD = 7.05)
4 Stopping ($\bar{x} = 3.70$; SD = 4.85)
5 Gliding ($\bar{x} = 0$)

For combinations of two processes, conspiring and feeding relationships were considered in the SIWI and SFWF positions. In both positions FLOSS for the feeding processes were higher than for the conspiring. While new homophony was produced as a function of two processes entering a process combination, it was also investigated whether the rank ordering of the FLOSS for the combinations of processes could be predicted on the basis of additive FLOSS-values for the respective single processes. To examine this, Spearman's correlation coefficients were calculated for feeding and conspiring processes and their corresponding additive FLOSS values as determined on the basis of the results for the single processes. Both coefficient values were above 0.9, which indicates a high correlation. Thus, the functional consequences of two processes operating in the particular combinations studied can be estimated on the basis of the additive FLOSS values for the respective single processes.

IMPLICATIONS FOR PHONOLOGICAL ASSESSMENT

The main goal of phonological assessment is to determine if there is a phonological disorder (Stoel-Gammon and Dunn, 1985). This is done by comparing the child's system with the adult target and with a developmental norm. This enables one to map out the contrastive and combinatory possibilities in the child's system and indicate any deviations from a norm. Having done this, treatment goals are formulated to bring the child's system in line with an adult and/or developmental norm. A different approach to assessment considers 'the communicative implications of the disordered speech patterns' in terms of 'the actual and implied failures to signal intended meanings unambiguously through the lack of adequate phonological contrasts' (Grunwell, 1987: 269). Having decided that a disorder exists, determining what the potential consequences of that disorder are for the child functioning as a communicator and improving the functional potential of the phonological system can provide some principled guidelines for the planning of specific treatment goals. Until recently (Leinonen, 1987, 1988), determining the functional (in)adequacy of children's phonological system has been largely speculative. Phonological assessment procedures attempting to serve this purpose have indicated variability, optionality, idiosyncracy, persistance, developmental deviance and frequency of phonological processes as possible indices of communicative inadequacy (e.g. Weiner, 1979; Hodson, 1980; Ingram, 1981; Grunwell, 1985). A further assessment goal serving this purpose is to determine the actual or potential homophony resulting from the contrastively restricted system. It remains to be shown how these relate to the communicative inadequacy (in the broad sense of the term) of a system. The measure and concept of FLOSS described in this chapter provides a more principled means of assessing the adequacy of children's disordered phonological systems in terms of their potential for homophony.

Work is currently in progress to develop an assessment protocol for assessing the functional adequacy of children's contrastively restricted phonological systems in terms of the concept and measure of FLOSS. Although this is incomplete, we can make some general observations on some of the main features of such a procedure.

The starting point is the identification of the phonological contrasts which are lacking from the child's phonological system. This can be done either with reference to a contrastive assessment such as Grunwell (1985) or in terms of a phonological process analysis. Keeping in line with the discussion thus far, I shall consider only assessment based on phonological process analysis here. I shall not, however, consider the general characteristics of process analyses or their advantages and disadvantages here (see Grunwell, 1987).

The first step is to identify the phonological processes operative in the child's speech and to determine which contrasts are consequently lacking in the phonological system. In doing this, it is necessary to work with processes rather than whole process categories (see above) in order to capture the possibility of processes across process categories conspiring (e.g. stopping /s–t/ and fronting /k–t/). It is also essential to identify interaction of processes which produce a particular lexical realization rather than treat co-occurring processes as separate processes (see Ingram, 1981; Grunwell, 1985, 1987). If the target /speis/ was realized as /beis/, cluster reduction of /sp–p/ and voicing of /p–b/ can be said to co-occur (or interact) in the word-initial position to produce the child realization. Failing to identify that these two processes enter a feeding relationship and thus treating these as separate processes would misrepresent the contrasts lacking from the system (i.e. not /sp–p/ and /p–b/ but /sp–b/ and /p–b/). Such failure would also obscure the assessment of the potential functional consequences of the system.

Having identified the processes present in the child's speech, the next step is to categorize them in terms of the functional motivations outlined above. Figure 5.1 represents the kinds of decisions involved in this categorization. First, it is necessary to determine whether the processes involve target-realization pairs which conflate or do not conflate phonological contrasts in the ambient language. Second, within the 'conflating' and 'non-conflating' groups of processes, it is decided whether the processes are conspiring or non-conspiring. Third, the non-conflating processes which are conspiring are divided into conspiring 'proper' and conspiring via feeding. This is also done for the conflating processes, for which also the non-conspiring processes are classified further. These are categorized as single

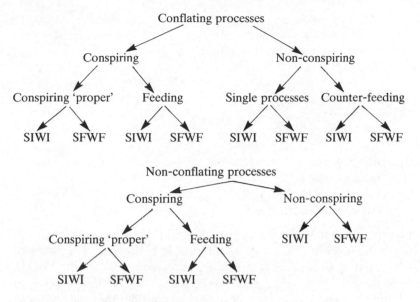

Figure 5.1 Categorization of processes

processes 'proper' or those entering a counter-feeding relationship. It is not necessary to draw this distinction for the non-conspiring processes which do not conflate contrasts since they have no potential for homophony. For all the processes it is also noted whether the processes operate in the SIWI or the SFWF places in structure.

To illustrate this, let us consider the following hypothetical set of processes. While, for exemplificatory purposes, it is clearer to work on a small hypothetical set, the procedure lends itself comfortably to larger process sets based on the analysis of real data samples.

SIWI:
Cluster reduction sk–k
Fronting k–t
Stopping s–t
Stopping s–t
↓
Voicing   t–d
Voicing t–d
Stopping v–b
Voicing p–b
Idiosyncratic k–x

SFWF:
Final consonant deletion t–0
Final consonant deletion s–0
Stopping z–d
        ↓
Devoicing d–t
Devoicing b–p
Devoicing   g–k
        ↓
Idiosyncratic   k–x
Idiosyncratic k–x
Glottal replacement g–?
Glottal replacement p–?

Figure 5.2 summarizes the categorization of these processes according to the functional motivations outlined in Figure 5.1. The potential
functional consequences can then be estimated by calculating FLOSS
values and/or by relying on the predictive devices discussed above. In
addition to these indices, it is necessary to consider the consistency of
occurrence of the phonological processes in the data sample in order
to reflect the potential functional implications of specific phonological systems more realistically. One process occurrence out of ten
possible ones is likely to have less detrimental implications for the
communicative adequacy of the phonological system than ten out of
ten possible occurrences. Consistency of process occurrences can be
measured as a ratio of the number of times a process or process
relationship occurs to the number of possible occurrences. How
precisely this information will be incorporated into estimating functional adequacy remains to be studied further.

IMPLICATIONS FOR THE PLANNING OF TREATMENT GOALS

One goal of phonological assessment is to generate suggestions for
specific treatment goals (Stoel-Gammon and Dunn, 1985). The
assessment of the functional adequacy of children's phonological
systems has direct implications for the planning of treatment goals. It
is reasonable to assume that homophony has to be kept to a tolerable
level in a lexical system for adequate linguistic and communicative
skills. Thus, elimination of those phonological processes from a
child's speech which have the greatest potential for homophony (e.g.
Leonard, 1985) is a well-motivated treatment goal.

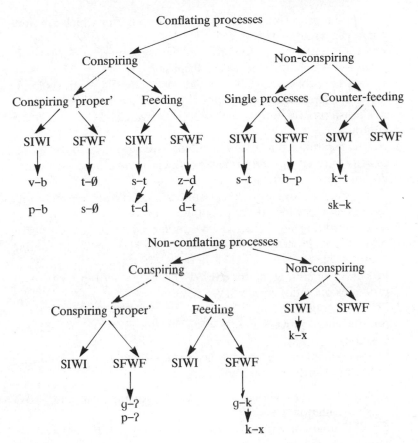

Figure 5.2 Example of categorization of processes

On the basis of the present discussion and the results of the study described above, specific suggestions for the planning of remedial goals can be made. Starting from the more general guidelines and working to the more specific the following 'orders of priority' can be inferred:

1 Processes which have potential for homophony (including multiple homophony) have priority over processes which cannot produce any homophony.
2 Processes which have potential for multiple homophony have priority over processes which have no potential for multiple homophony.

3 Conspiring processes have priority over processes which are non-conspiring (single processes).
4 Processes entering a feeding relationship merit priority over processes which are otherwise conspiring.
5 Conspiring processes which conflate phonological contrasts in the ambient language have priority over conspiring process relationships which involve processes which do not conflate contrasts.
6 Non-conspiring contrasts which conflate contrasts merit equal priority with conspiring processes which involve processes which do not conflate contrasts.
7 Excepting 6 (above), processes conflating contrasts merit priority over processes which do not conflate contrasts.
8 Non-conspiring processes which conflate contrasts merit priority over such processes when they enter a counter-feeding relationship.
9 Processes operating in the SFWF position merit priority over processes operating in the SIWI position.
10 Processes operating in the SFWF and SIWI positions merit priority over processes operating in the SFWW and SIWW positions.
11 If one chooses to work on whole process categories the following orders of priority can be suggested:

SIWI: fronting > gliding > prevocalic   voicing > stopping > WI cluster reduction
SFWF: final-consonant deletion > fronting > WF devoicing > stopping > gliding

These general guidelines provide a means of estimating functional consequences of contrastively restricted phonological systems. For more specific guidelines, one can utilize ready-calculated FLOSS values (Leinonen, 1987, 1988). As was discussed above, FLOSS values for single processes can be added together to indicate the functional consequences of processes which are non-conspiring and otherwise incompatible with new homophony. Also, the results indicated that FLOSS of combinations of two (and possibly more) processes can be estimated on the basis of the respective additive FLOSS values.

These priorities are theoretically motivated for elimination of homophony in children's phonological systems. This is one potential approach to remedial planning and needs to be interrelated to other potential influences bearing upon the communicative inadequacy of a disordered phonological system. As such, these priorities as potential guidelines for remediation do not exist in a vacuum. For instance, a child may have difficulty in producing word-final segments altogether and this would influence the planning of homophony reduction. Speech-language clinicians have the experience and knowledge to incorporate such considerations into the above suggestions on an individual basis.

CONCLUSIONS

While the assessment of the functional adequacy of children's phonological systems is a well-motivated enterprise, many details which would promote its applicability to the clinical management of phonological disorders in children remain to be worked out. There are two main considerations which are to be addressed next: first, the mechanics of the assessment and the planning of remedial goals need to be refined, and possibly simplified, on the basis of analysis of real data from phonologically disordered children; second, how does functional adequacy of a phonological system relate to its communicative adequacy? Being able to make the assessment of the functional adequacy more communicatively orientated would render the concept more clinically useful. Work is currently in progress to address these issues.

The concept and measure of FLOSS also lends itself to the study of child phonology *per se*. For instance, it can be studied whether FLOSS correlates with the order and progress of phonological change in developing phonological systems. Is there evidence for the development of contrasts with high FLOSS before those with low FLOSS? Similarly, the notion of FLOSS can be valuable for exploring possible homophony avoidance. Do children's developing phonologies structure themselves so that homophony in lexical systems is minimized? Investigations such as these would not only enhance our knowledge of phonological development but would also feed into clinical management of phonological disorders in children.

APPENDIX

The phonological processes included in the study

1 WI cluster reduction
   pl–p; bl–b; pr–p; br–b; tr–t; dr–d; kr–k; gr–g; kl–k; gl–g; kw–k; fr–f; fl–f; θr–θ; sp–p; st–t; sk–k; sm–m; sn–n; sl–l; sw–s; spl–p; spr–p; skr–k; skw–k; str–t.

2 Stopping of fricatives and affricates
   f–p; v–b; θ–t; ð–d; s–t; z–d; ʃ–t; ʒ–d; tʃ–t; dʒ–d.
3 Fronting
   k–t; g–d; ŋ–n.
4 Gliding of liquids
   l–w; l–j; r–w; r–j.
5 Prevocalic voicing
   p–b; t–d; k–g; f–v; θ–ð; ʃ–ʒ; s–z; tʃ–dʒ.
6 WF devoicing
   b–p; d–t; g–k; v–f; ð–θ; ʒ–ʃ; z–s; dʒ–tʃ.
7 Final-consonant deletion
   n–0; m–0; p–0; b–0; t–0; d–0; k–0; g–0; f–0; v–0; θ–0; ð–0; s–0;
   z–0; ʃ–0; ʒ–0; tʃ–0; dʒ–0.
8 Glottal replacement
   p–ʔ; b–ʔ; t–ʔ; d–ʔ; s–ʔ; z–ʔ; tʃ–ʔ; dʒ–ʔ.

REFERENCES

Burrough, G. E. R. (1957) *A Study of the Vocabulary of Young Children*, Edinburgh: Oliver & Boyd.
Connolly, J. H. (1980) 'An explanatory role of linguistics in relation to speech therapy', *Belfast Working Papers in Language and Linguistics* 4: 85–98.
Connolly, J. H. (1984) 'Speech intelligibility; a clinical linguistic perspective', unpublished paper, Leicester Polytechnic, UK.
Grunwell, P. (1985) *Phonological Assessment of Child Speech*, Windsor: NFER–Nelson.
Grunwell, P. (1987) *Clinical Phonology*, 2nd ed, London: Croom Helm.
Hodson, B. W. (1980) *The Assessment of Phonological Processes*, Danville, IL: Interstate.
Ingram, D. (1975) 'Surface contrast in children's speech', *Journal of Child Language* 2: 287–92.
Ingram, D. (1981) *Procedures for the Phonological Assessment of Children's Language*, Baltimore: University Park Press.
Kiparsky, P. (1968) 'Linguistic universals and linguistic change', in E. Bach and R. T. Harms (eds) *Universals in Linguistic Theory*, London: Holt, Rinehart & Winston; 170–202.
Kiparsky, P. and Menn, L. (1977) 'On the acquisition of phonology', in J. MacNamara (ed.) *Language Learning and Thought*, London: Academic Press, 47–78.
Leinonen, E. (1987) 'Assessing the functional adequacy of children's phonological systems', unpublished PhD thesis, Leicester Polytechnic, UK.
Leinonen, E. (1988) 'Assessing the functional adequacy of children's phonological systems', *Clinical Linguistics and Phonetics* 2(4): 257–70.
Leonard, L. B. (1985) 'Unusual and subtle phonological behaviour in the speech of phonologically disordered children', *Journal of Speech and Hearing Disorders* 50: 4–13.

Line, P. (1987) 'An investigation of auditory distance', unpublished M Phil. thesis, Leicester Polytechnic, UK.

Newton, K. (1971) 'Ordering paradoxes in phonology', *Journal of Linguistics* 7: 31–53.

Shriberg, L. D. and Kwiatkowski, J. (1980) *Natural Process Analysis: a Procedure for Phonological Analysis of Continuous Speech Samples*, New York: Wiley.

Smith, B. R. and Leinonen, E. (forthcoming) *Clinical Pragmatics*, London: Chapman & Hall.

Stampe, D. (1979) *A Dissertation on Natural Phonology*, New York: Garland.

Stoel-Gammon, C. and Dunn, C. (1985) *Normal and Disordered Phonology in Children*, Baltimore: University Park Press.

Weiner, F. F. (1979) *Phonological Process Analysis*, Baltimore: University Park Press.

6 Facilitating intelligibility: assessment, therapy and consideration across languages

Barbara Williams Hodson

The phonological approach that is described in this chapter was designed for highly unintelligible American English-speaking children. Many of the principles that have been effective for this approach can be used to design phonological assessment and remediation procedures for other languages. The approach has been adapted for use with Spanish-speaking children in Mexico, Colombia and Puerto Rico, as well as in the United States and phonological assessment instruments have been developed for Navajo-speaking children and for children from the Philippines who speak Tagalog.

Clinical hypotheses have been developed and tested while working with approximately two hundred clients in a university clinic. The approach is being used successfully in hospitals, clinics and schools to expedite intelligibility gains in children with severe/profound speech disorders throughout the United States and Canada. The primary difference between this remediation approach and phoneme-orientated articulation programmes is that *cycles* are used to facilitate the development of phonological patterns.

Cycles are time periods during which *all* phonological patterns in need of remediation are facilitated in succession. Phonemes within the phonological patterns (e.g., voiceless final stops for the pattern of final consonants) are used to facilitate emergence of the respective patterns. Phonological patterns are *recycled* during ensuing cycles, and *complexity* is increased gradually during each succeeding cycle via incorporating production-practice words with more difficult phonetic environments and also by grouping phonemes within target patterns.

Some cycles are five or six weeks in length; others may be as long as fifteen or sixteen weeks. Usually three to six cycles involving approximately thirty to forty hours of a speech-language pathologist's time (sixty minutes per week) are required for a phonologically disordered client to become intelligible with this approach.

PROCEDURES

Assessment

The Assessment of Phonological Processes – Revised (Hodson, 1986a) was designed for highly unintelligible English-speaking children, and the Assessment of Phonological Processes – Spanish (Hodson, 1986b) was developed for Spanish-speaking children with severe/profound speech disorders. Objects are used to elicit spontaneous naming responses. Speech deviations are recorded at the time of utterance via narrow phonetic transcription. In addition, the child's sample is recorded on audiotape to be replayed later for transcription verification. Language samples are also recorded, but most of the connected-speech utterances during the initial assessment session cannot be analysed because of the lack of intelligible words. The connected-speech samples are useful for comparisons over time as the child becomes more intelligible.

The phonological assessment instruments (English and Spanish) were designed to meet the unique needs of each language. The Spanish instrument is *not* a translation of the English version. Both instruments were field-tested on intelligible and unintelligible subjects to identify both normal and disordered phonological processes in the respective languages (Hodson *et al.*, 1984).

The phonological assessment instruments were designed to meet the following criteria:

1   Phonological assessment results indicate not only whether there is a disorder, but also the severity of the disorder.
2   Results of phonological assessment provide a direction for planning remediation.
3   Scores following intervention provide accountability measures.
4   Administration time (contact time with child) does not exceed twenty minutes; analysis time does not exceed sixty minutes.

Selecting target patterns phonemes

It is important to initiate a highly unintelligible client's phonological remediation programme with a pattern for which the client has 'readiness'. This does not mean that it is appropriate to start with patterns that the child already produces. Rather, the clinician should select from the client's phonological deficiencies the pattern that is most stimulable so that the child can experience immediate success. The next most stimulable deficient pattern is targeted second and so on until *all* primary patterns that are deficient have been stimulated during *each* cycle, and all patterns, that have not yet begun to emerge in conversational speech by the beginning of each ensuing cycle are recycled.

The ordering of phonological patterns for presentation within a cycle depends on the individual child. However, findings obtained from clinical and developmental phonology research (e.g. Ingram, 1975; Hodson and Paden, 1981; Stoel-Gammon and Dunn, 1985; Preisser *et al.*, 1988) provide guidelines.

Most preschool children sequence at least two syllables. Two- and three-syllable compound words, preferably with equal stress, are appropriate targets for children who have not yet learned to produce syllables in sequences. The emphasis during this time is on the appropriate number of syllables rather than on specific consonants. It has been observed that as children learn to sequence two and three syllables in their phonological systems, they typically also develop two-word utterances in their expressive language.

Prevocalic anterior nasals, stops and the labial glide do not often need to be targeted. If a child completely lacks any of these phoneme classes, however, the labial and alveolar phonemes within these early developing classes would be appropriate targets (sixty minutes per each deficient phoneme in the designated pattern). Phonemes that the child is already producing should *not* be targeted even if they are produced inconsistently.

A third basic phonological pattern is final consonants. Word-final voiceless stops and/or word-final nasals (if lacking) are appropriate targets to help children develop the ability to close syllables. Voiced word-final obstruents should *not* be targets for highly unintelligible English-speaking children because their phonologically normal peers typically do not fully voice utterance-final obstruents (Hodson and Paden, 1981).

Occasionally, a child will produce final consonants in some words and initial consonants in others, but will lack CVC (initial and final consonants in the same word). Monosyllabic words containing the same initial and final consonant can be used to help a child learn that consonants can occur at the beginning and also at the end of the same word. (It must be remembered, of course, that many languages do not contain such words.)

If a child lacks either velar or alveolar stops because of *fronting* or *backing*, these classes should be evaluated next for readiness. However, some children experience considerable difficulty with these patterns, particularly word-initial velars. It may be necessary to delay production-practice for such children for a cycle until they are stimulable for velars.

Stridents and consonant sequences should be targeted during each cycle as well as any deficient patterns from lower developmental levels. It is preferable to target /s/ in consonant sequences rather than as singletons during early cycles because highly unintelligible children tend to produce /s/-plus-stop combinations when attempts are made by the clinician to elicit singleton /s/.

The /l/ and /r/ phonemes should also be stimulated during *each* cycle; however, they usually are the last phonemes targeted per cycle. The goal for early cycles is to develop awareness of /l/ and /r/ and to suppress substitution processes (e.g., *gliding, stopping*, rather than for the child to produce perfect /l/ and /r/. If an appropriate foundation is laid during initial cycles, /l/ and /r/ begin to *emerge* during the period that the other phonological patterns are being generalized into spontaneous utterances.

It is recommended that each phoneme within a pattern be targeted for approximately *sixty minutes* before moving on to the next phoneme in that pattern and then on to other phonological patterns. Furthermore, it is desirable to provide *two* or more phoneme targets within a pattern before progressing on to the next pattern. Generally, only one phonological pattern should be presented during any one session, with the exception of stridency and consonant sequences, which are targeted in /s/ clusters for the first few cycles.

Phonemes serve as a 'means to an end' in cycles, rather than an end in themselves. Phonemes are *not* taught to a preselected criterion (e.g. 90 per cent). Rather, carefully chosen production-practice words with the session's target phoneme(s) are utilized to help the child develop new auditory and kinesthetic images for the purpose of eventual *self-monitoring*. The first cycle lays the *phonological foundation* and allows the child to experience immediate and tangible success on carefully selected production-practice words. Carry-over to other words is not expected until a later cycle.

Selecting production-practice words

It is recommended that words (rather than nonsense syllables) be used for production practice. Whenever possible, monosyllabic words with facilitative phonetic environments should be selected during the first two cycles so that the child can experience some immediate success. Words that contain phonemes produced at the same *place* of articulation as the substitute phoneme should be avoided during early cycles, and care should be taken to reduce opportunities for assimilation effects.

Words for which actual objects can be incorporated are desirable for preschool children. In addition, 'action' words should be used to add another dimension. It is important that production-practice words be appropriate for each child's vocabulary level and linguistic community.

Facilitating development of awareness of phonological patterns

The purpose of production practice in this approach is *not* to establish a motor pattern. Rather, it is to help the child develop a new *Kinaesthetic image* for self-monitoring purposes. At the same time, it is imperative to help the child develop auditory awareness of the pattern. Auditory bombardment with *minimal amplification* is provided for a few minutes at the beginning and again at the end of *every* phonological session.

Most children with highly unintelligible speech demonstrate relatively poor listening skills, especially for their own speech. They seem to rely solely on their own inaccurate kinesthetic images which 'feel right' at the time, and they tend to ignore or negate auditory feedback for their inaccurate productions. Many adults have experienced being corrected by a child after saying a word exactly like the child. This correction is typically followed by the child's repetition of the identical error production. Unintelligible children do not seem to *hear* their own speech. Combining a limited amount of production practice with amplified auditory training during each session seems to help children improve their self-monitoring skills. The amplifier is also used during times when a child seems to be having a great deal of difficulty with a production.

This remediation approach should *not* be used without incorporating amplification. Children respond differently when the listening list is presented with amplification than when the clinician simply says the words loudly without amplification. One problem that often accompanies the reading of words without amplification is that clinicians tend to exaggerate their models, particularly for /s/. It is imperative that a soft, precise /s/ be modelled for two reasons: young children tend to 'overproduce' what has been modelled, with the result being distorted sibilants; the second reason is that the more precise /s/ production enables the child to experience a more definitive kinesthetic image for matching purposes.

Structure of the remediation session

The following format has been used in our university clinic and adapted for other professional settings.

1   The child reviews the preceding session's production-practice word cards. If target patterns are being changed, the cards from the preceding week are set aside until a later cycle. They can be reused, and new words can be added during ensuing cycles to increase complexity. If the phoneme target for this session is for the same target pattern as the last session, both sets of cards can be incorporated into some production-practice activities for the current session.

2   The clinician provides auditory bombardment with *slight amplification* for a couple of minutes. The child listens through a headset while the clinician reads the session's listening list of approximately fifteen words that contain the target pattern. The child must *not* say these words; rather he or she must listen attentively. The clinician may also demonstrate the error and contrast it with the target while using the amplifier.

3   The child draws/colours (or pastes on) three to five pictures of carefully selected production-practice words (controlled for phonetic environment) on 5 × 8 inch index cards. The child says the word prior to making the picture so that the clinician can check for the appropriateness/difficulty of each word. The clinician writes the word on the card so that the adults will be able to identify the child's pictures.

4   The child participates in *experiential-play* production-practice activities. He or she names the picture incorporating the target pattern for the day in order to 'take a turn'. The clinician provides models and/or tactual cues as needed so that the child achieves 100 per cent success on the target pattern for these carefully selected production-practice words. The clinician provides opportunities for spontaneous conversation during each session in order to observe when phonological patterns are beginning to emerge.

5   The clinician *probes* for *stimulability* for the next session's target phoneme within the selected target pattern. The most stimulable phoneme within the pattern is selected to be the target for the following session.

6   The clinician repeats amplified auditory training. The same listening list of words that was used earlier in the session is again read to the child.

7   The parent (or school aide) participates in a two-minutes per day home (or school) programme. An adult reads the listening list

and the child names the picture cards of production-practice words once a day.

Remediation activities

Experiential-play activities (e.g. fishing, bowling) provide motivation for young children. It is especially beneficial to incorporate pragmatically appropriate activities; furthermore, it is recommended that some of the remediation activities occur outside the clinician's room.

The use of *minimal-pair* words is excellent for children who have sufficient skills to experience success (Tyler *et al.*, 1987) and for languages that have appropriate minimal-pair words. Explanations of minimal-pair differences can be provided even if the child is not ready to produce the contrasting words. During the final cycles, the use of minimal pairs can be extremely effective in helping children recognize the semantic differences of the two productions.

The number of activities varies from session to session. In general, our student clinicians average one activity for every seven or eight minutes. The same activities can be used week after week. Clinicians are advised to change to the next activity *before* children lose interest, even if they wish to continue certain activities.

Student clinicians in our phonology programme do not count and chart errors. Inaccurate productions do not help children develop appropriate new kinesthetic images. Instead, the clinicians use their skills to provide sufficient cues so that clients can produce targets appropriately. For instance, clinicians typically provide models and tactual cues (e.g. drawing a finger up the child's arm for /s/ and tapping for a /t/ in an /s/-cluster word) at the beginning of sessions. The cues are decreased as the client gains facility.

For older clients who can read, a short period of *oral reading* focusing on the session's target patterns is beneficial. The reading material for this activity should be at a level that is *lower* than the child's current reading ability so that attention can be directed towards the phonological pattern rather than on reading skills.

Some children may need to start one step below production practice. For clients who lack stimulability or who are unwilling to participate in production-practice activities (e.g. two-year-olds) it may be best to provide *focused auditory input* during the first cycle. The deficient patterns are stimulated by presenting one new phoneme (within a target pattern) per week. The child participates in activities and listens, but production is not required during this cycle. The clinician talks about the selected objects and incorporates activities related to the week's target phoneme. All of the deficient patterns are presented in this manner (auditorily) for a cycle. Production-practice activities are incorporated during the second and later cycles (i.e., after the child demonstrates sufficient readiness).

DISCUSSION

All remediation approaches (and also maturation) appear to help children improve speech (Ingram, 1983); however, times required for a child to achieve intelligibility vary considerably from one approach to another. Phoneme-orientated approaches that target one phoneme at a time for several months until a criterion (e.g. 90 per cent) is reached are generally appropriate for a child who has only two or three speech-sound errors. However, phoneme-orientated approaches have proved to be very time-consuming for children with extensive speech errors. Five years or more of therapy are typically required before a child with a severe/profound speech disorder becomes intelligible via phoneme-orientated approaches. Children need to become intelligible as quickly as possible, especially if they are trying to read and spell (Hodson *et al.* 1989).

The longest period of remediation time required for cognitively normal children with profound phonological disorders to become intelligible via the cycles approach, which involves facilitating patterns rather than perfecting individual phonemes, has been eighteen months (approximately sixty hours of remediation time). Most preschool children require less than a year of remediation. The cycles approach more closely approximates the way in which normal phonological development occurs than does teaching phonemes one by one to a particular criterion level (Ingram, 1986).

The cycles remediation approach has been adapted effectively for use with children with developmental dyspraxia (Hodson and Paden, 1983) and with repaired cleft palates (Hodson *et al.* 1991). This approach has also been used successfully for children with moderate-to-severe hearing impairments (Garret, 1986). Furthermore, the approach has been adapted for use with children in mentally retarded classrooms. Time allotments, however, have been doubled for mentally retarded children. Each phoneme per pattern is targeted two hours rather than sixty minutes, and approximately three years are required before substantial intelligibility gains are observed. Mentally retarded children need a comprehensive phonological remediation programme even more than normal children because they lack the cognitive abilities necessary to integrate isolated phoneme parts.

SOME CONSIDERATIONS FOR OTHER LANGUAGES

The cycles approach has not been used extensively with languages other than English. Assessment instruments that identify critical phonological processes need to be developed in other languages. The three phonological processes that have most distinguished unintelligible Spanish- and English-speaking children from their phonologically normal peers are consonant-sequence reduction, stridency deletion and deviations involving /l/ and /r/ phonemes (Hodson *et al.* 1984). Every unintelligible child tested in Spanish and English thus far has evidenced these three error patterns to some extent.

Final-consonant deletion and velar deviations have also been prevalent in utterances of many unintelligible children, but these latter phonological processes have not been evidenced by all unintelligible children. Each phonologically disordered child is an individual, and no two children have had identical phonologies; none the less, commonalities have been observed across children and for two languages (Spanish and English).

The first step for any language is to develop and test assessment instruments that focus on unintelligible phonological processes. Disordered processes must be separated from developmental and dialectal patterns. The second step is to develop and test comprehensive phonological remediation approaches. The cycles approach can be adapted for languages other than English. Target phonological patterns and target words need to be identified, and aspects of each language must be considered. Cross-linguistic research can yield important information about normal and disordered phonological development which will undoubtedly have both theoretical and practical implications for child phonology.

REFERENCES

Garret, R. (1986) 'A phonologically based speech-improvement classroom program for hearing-impaired students', unpublished manuscript, San Diego State University.

Hodson, B. (1986a) *Assessment of Phonological Processes – Revised,* Austin Tx: Pro-Ed.

Hodson, B. (1986b) *Assessment of Phonological Processes – Spanish,* San Diego: Los Amigos.

Hodson, B. and Paden, E. (1981) 'Phonological processes which characterize unintelligible and intelligible speech in early childhood', *Journal of Speech and Hearing Disorders* 46: 369–73.

Hodson, B. and Paden, E. (1991) *Targeting Intelligible Speech: a Phonological Approach to Remediation,* 2nd ed., Austin Tx: Pro-Ed.

Hodson, B., Nonomum, C., and Zappin, M. (1989) 'Phonological disorders: Impact on academic performance', *Seminars in Speech and Language* 10: 252–9.

Hodson, B., Becker, M., Diamond, F. and Meza, P. (1984) 'Phonological analysis of unintelligible children's utterances: English and Spanish', in G. Nathan and M. Winters (eds) *Occasional Papers in Linguistics: the Uses of Phonology*, Carbondale: Southern Illinois University Press: 61–7.

Hodson, B., Chin, L., Redmond, B. and Simpson, R. (1983) 'Phonological evaluation and remediation of speech deviations of a child with a repaired cleft palate: a case study', *Journal of Speech and Hearing Disorders* 48: 93–8.

Ingram, D. (1975) *Phonological Disability in Children*, New York: Elsevier.

Ingram, D. (1983) 'Case studies of phonological disability', *Topics in Language Disorders* 3: viii.

Ingram, D. (1986) 'Explanation and phonological remediation', *Child Language Teaching and Therapy* 2: 1–19.

Preisser, D., Hodson, B. and Paden, E. (1988) 'Developmental phonology: 18–29 months', *Journal of Speech and Hearing Disorders* 53: 125–30.

Stoel-Gammon, C. and Dunn, C. (1985) *Normal and Disordered Phonology in Children*, Austin: Pro-Ed.

Tyler, A., Edwards, M. and Saxman, J. (1987) 'Clinical application of two phonologically based treatment procedures', *Journal of Speech and Hearing Disorders* 52: 393–409.

7 Input training in phonological disorder: a case discussion

Susanna Evershed Martin

This chapter aims to summarize what, in the author's appreciation, is the current state of thinking and practice in the United Kingdom in the management of children with marked disorders of speech output. A single case is presented around which a number of unresolved issues are discussed. Emphasis is placed on the position of 'input training' in the remediation of such disorders.

INTRODUCTION

In any field of endeavour when a radical innovation of thinking occurs, the new order which is as a result introduced is hailed as possessing the truth, and the old order that it supersedes is discarded. Later, as the new philosophy matures and is moderated in the light of experience, it not infrequently proves to be incapable of fulfilling early promise, and a reappraisal of the old order of thinking can reveal its displaced value. Such is the path of history in the study, assessment and management of children with developmental disorders of speech. Radical changes in the fashion of theoretical description, assessment of disorder and strategies for remediation have occurred (and will doubtless continue to occur in future) in many areas of speech pathology, and is clearly evidenced in the last twenty years in the study of what are now generally referred to as 'phonological disorders'. Since the early 1970s the emphasis has moved from the articulatory to the phonological. Disorders which involved any failure of speech output were earlier described as *articulatory* or *articulation disorders*, regardless of whether the failure lay within the area of central phonological language functioning or within lower phonetic levels of articulation (though the term 'functional articulation disorder' was sometimes used). With the publication of Ingram's book *Phonological Disability in Children* (1976) clinical linguists included the possibility of speech output being disordered, not at the articulatory level, but at the level of central cortical representation of speech-sound patterning, and the terms *phonological disorder* and *phonological disability* entered the vocabulary. Workers in the field accepted the new insights which this change of emphasis engendered with such enthusiasm and interest that by the early 1980s the articulatory dimension had been almost entirely lost. Thus a 'pendulum swing' (Grunwell, 1985a) had occurred; the ubiquitous use of *articulatory* descriptions had given way to the almost exclusive use of *phonological* descriptions.

DESCRIPTION AND EXPLANATION

More recently, Grunwell (1985a), Harris and Cottam (1985), Hawkins (1985), Hewlett (1985) and Milroy (1985) have sought to redress the balance between phonological and articulatory approaches, acknowledging the need to retain a clear distinction between disorders arising from breakdown in phonological processing and those which arise at the phonoarticulatory level. Grunwell (1985a), in a clear exposition of the discussion in train, highlights the need to distinguish between the analysis of language as either 'a systematic *description* of the observed patterns produced' or as 'a psycholinguistic *explanation* of the actual processes involved in a person's production of speech patterns'. In other words, the term *phonological disorder* is potentially ambiguous. In one sense it may be applied, subsequent to analysis, to imply that the *speech patterns* lack contrastive, and hence communicative, power. In the other sense, the term is used to distinguish the disorder as phonological *in origin*, that is that the *speaker* lacks the phonological capacity to utilize contrastive, and hence communicative, power, from one which is articulatory or phonetic, where the disability lies in the translation of unaffected phonological capacity into matching articulations. The two analyses are described by Hewlett (1985) as being, in the first case, *data-orientated* – speech patterns are *described* as phonologically inadequate, and in the second *speaker-orientated* – an explanation of *why* speech patterns are disordered is provided, and aetiology is thereby specified.

PHONETIC AND PHONOLOGICAL APPROACHES IN REMEDIATION

An explanation or diagnosis of disorder is a highly desirable (though frequently elusive) prerequisite of treatment; if analysis stops at description of speech-output failure without seeking an explanation for that failure, then strategies in remediation cannot be tailored to individual needs, and nothing more than a 'general speech' approach can be taken. It must be assumed that, if a phonological explanation has been sought and found, then the therapy applied should be grounded in phonology; in the absence of articulatory failure, articulation therapy, though not harmful, clearly does not strike at the heart of the matter. Conversely, where mispronunciations arise from failure in the planning and execution of speech movement, to approach remediation 'phonologically', by, for example, minimal-pair confrontation, is to by-pass the child's paramount need for phonetic practice (i.e. articulation therapy), and to fail to acknowledge his or her intact phonological capacity.

In theory, then, it is important that both phonological and phonetic/articulatory factors are addressed in the assessment of disorder prior to treatment; remediation strategies are then directed towards the level of disorder identified as predominantly responsible for the breakdown in speech output. In practice, however, cases are frequently encountered where the explanation of disorder remains hard to identify; speech lacks contrastive power, that is it can be *described* as phonologically disordered, but no clear aetiology can be isolated, that is the explanation for disorder may be either phonological or articulatory, or a combination of both. This is most clearly seen in children whose speech is markedly unintelligible and yet who have no demonstrable organic deficit. Current practice suggests that a disorder may be interpreted as phonological in origin where no dyspraxia, dysarthria or vocal-tract anomaly can be demonstrated. If one or more of these can be shown to exist then it is fair to assume that an articulatory dimension is at least contributing to breakdown in speech acquisition. The dynamic interaction of the three articulatory levels, motor-planning, neuromuscular functioning and vocal-tract movement, to which these three disorders relate respectively, with the phonological level cannot, however, be ignored. Is it to be assumed that if a child exhibits symptoms of developmental articulatory dyspraxia (developmental apraxia of speech; see Jaffe, 1984) his or her *phonological* acquisition will proceed along normal lines? It would seem, rather, that the *experience* of age-appropriate articulatory skills contributes to 'correct' functioning and the normal progression in development of both phonology and its articulatory realization, which are intimately bound together. If phonology is thought of solely as dependent on articulation for its realization, the equal balance between phonological capacity and matched articulatory experience is overlooked. Once normal acquisition is complete (that is, in 'adult' phonology), then the model which assumes articulation to be the independent vehicle for phonology holds up to scrutiny, but during the process of acquisition the dynamic part which articulatory practice and experimentation play in establishing phonological patterns should not be ignored. If articulation and phonology develop independently, then it is hard to explain why babbling continues beyond the age of emergence of true speech, and why phonetic variability and experimentation remain a feature of early language acquisition. (See Fawcus, 1980 and Edwards, 1984, for further discussion of phonoarticulatory skills and phonology.)

It is important, then, in both assessment and remediation that the interaction of phonological and articulatory capacity is constantly kept in mind. This is most especially so in the type of case where no clear explanation of disorder emerges. Treatment in such cases should, by addressing itself to both articulation and phonology, aim to inform a clearer diagnosis. It is frequently impossible, especially in cases of marked unintelligibility, to attribute disorder to a specific cause. No professional, in such circumstances, can wait until cause has been established beyond doubt, but must, rather, start treatment. If both aspects of speech output are targeted in therapy, then the individual's interactions and progress in each aspect of training may serve to inform diagnosis more closely. Put simply: the remediation process itself is part of the diagnostic process, and assessment is continuous.

OUTPUT AND INPUT IN ASSESSMENT AND REMEDIATION

To address output levels as the point at which most assessment begins is not to suggest that input is ignored. To give a somewhat far-fetched example: no speech/language specialist would agree to set aside as irrelevant a 50dB bilateral hearing loss in a child with markedly disturbed patterns of speech! If there is any truth in models of speech and language functioning which emphasize the synergistic relationship between levels within output, as is suggested above, then this must be extended to include a balanced 'feed-back' *and* 'feed-forward' relationship between input and output. Whilst, however, audiology has come far in assessing different types of hearing loss, the intermediate level between auditory transmission (conductive and neural) and central language, that is, the level of auditory perception,

remains shrouded in mystery. Though a number of speech-discrimination tests exist (Wepman, 1958; Goldman *et al.*, 1970; Pronovost,
1974), it is by no means certain how useful these are in assessing
auditory perceptual skills. Bountress and Laderberg (1981) and
Bountress (1984) challenge the validity of results using these tests,
since conflicting results are obtained from their use. Though
researchers have attempted to throw light on this complex area, it has
to be acknowledged that the field has advanced little as far as clinical
applications are concerned. The therapist is still in much the same
position as in the 1960s and earlier, when the need to address perception in assessment was recognized, but with no certainty that the tools
available were particularly sensitive or informative. In 1957 Liberman
et al. published their study on categorical perception which has subsequently served as the model for research. The perceptual abilities of
infants has been extensively investigated: Eimas *et al.* (1971) showed
that babies as young as one month are able to perceive within the
same general categories as do adults. The relationship between
perception and production in individuals with both normal and disordered speech has been of interest to such as Williams (1974),
Locke and Kutz (1975), McReynolds *et al.* (1975), Borden (1980)
and Locke (1980a, 1980b). The observation has frequently been
made that children are able to perceive errors in the speech of others,
so that when their mispronunciations are echoed back to them they
protest, the so-called 'fis phenomenum' (Berko and Brown, 1960; see
also Grunwell, 1982), but apparently fail to note their own faulty
output. The explanation of such failure may be either that perception
of others is ahead of self-perception and/or production; or that the
child perceives his or her own speech in a different way than do
adults, the perceptual boundaries for phonemic contrasts not
matching closely that of adults. A third possibility is that perception is
in some way 'distorted' or 'confused' by lack of productive ability; the
child cannot be clear about perceiving his or her own mispronunciations until production is sufficiently refined that it ceases to 'inter-
fere' with perception. Thus, as Borden and Harris (1980: 199) sur-
mise 'perception not only aids production, but the mastery of the
production of speech sounds is viewed as an aid to the child in his
effort to discriminate the sounds of the speech of others'.

Great difficulties are encountered in identifying the processes
involved in speech perception and, as is suggested above, despite
continuing research, the speech therapist faced with a child with
unintelligible speech has yet to find readily available assessment aids
which can throw clear light on perceptual functioning. Borden and

Harris's conclusion would, however, appear to have a ready and important application in the remediation of speech disorders, and further supports the view that the phonological and articulatory levels cannot be treated as independent in the management of such disorders, since perception must be prerequisite to the acquisition of phonological capacity.

A THREE-DIMENSIONAL APPROACH TO REMEDIATION

If it is accepted that a balance between all levels of speech and language processing acting interdependently must exist for speech to develop normally, then it is logical to suppose that remediation which treats as independent any single level of functioning is inadequate. Whilst, as mentioned above, it is desirable to attempt to isolate articulatory, phonological or perceptual breakdown, it is frequently not possible so to do. When clear diagnosis is possible, in, say, the case of a child with cleft palate, articulation therapy is seen not as standing alone, but as the means to the end which incorporates improved and adapted speech movements in the child's phonology and perception of speech (both inter- and intrapersonal). Whilst the boundaries between perception, phonology and articulation are by no means fully clarified, it is suggested that in every case of output failure therapy should address all three. In cases where aetiology remains obscure, the clinician may ensure, by including training in all three areas, that allowance is made for all the possible contributory factors. Whilst it may, in other cases, be possible to isolate a predominant cause whilst dismissing others as less dynamic in speech inadequacy, the clinician has to bear in mind potential difficulties involved in incorporating altered perception and/or articulation into phonological usage, or conversely of realizing perceived phonological contrast in articulation.

The recent fashion that describes (but possibly fails to explain) disorders as phonological has led to therapies which suggest an immediate attack at the phonological level by using techniques such as minimal-pair confrontation (eg. Weiner, 1981), whilst by-passing articulation and perception *per se*. This is not to suggest that those who recommend such treatment methods do not first ensure that the phonological contrast or process being addressed can be perceived. But if, for example, the target for remediation is to modify the process of stopping of fricatives, then minimal pairs such as *fight/bite, sock/tock* may be presented and the child is first asked to discriminate between them. If he or she is able to do so, is it to be assumed perception is not of importance? If he or she is able in isolation to produce [s], can the articulatory level be by-passed? Objections must arise; first, in identifying one of a minimal pair, a 'maximally aided' situation is present, nor is such perception typical of the normal situation in which speech is acquired. No child, when learning the phonology of his or her language, is given such specific information. I do not say to my child: 'Put on your sock, not your tock, rock, lock, etc.' He needs repeated and 'unaided' experience of input to identify sounds from the wide spectrum of incoming information. Second, the ability to produce in isolation a single speech-sound is only tenuously linked to the complex process involved in the rapid and generalized use of that sound in language. Again, in normal development children are observed to produce accurately in speech play and babble sounds which are not yet part of their phonologies.

Of the many therapy approaches reported in recent years, Hodson and Paden's (1983) is one which addresses the needs of speech-disordered children by including as essential both input and output. Furthermore, the 'cyclic' nature of their programme reflects the gradual nature of phonological acquisition. In what follows, the progress of a single child is presented, for whom an eclectic approach was adopted, but whose therapy included a heavy component of input training, involving techniques akin to those recommended by Hodson and Paden (1983).

INITIAL ASSESSMENT

M was first seen aged 4 years 5 months. She was, for the most part, unintelligible; it was sometimes possible to understand short utterances, but these were usually supported by environmental clues. In longer utterances it was impossible to understand more than the occasional word. She was rather withdrawn, preferring to rely on her mother or siblings to speak for her; her lack of willingness to communicate was, in the light of the grossly disordered nature of her speech, hardly surprising, since she must have constantly encountered her own communicative inadequacy. She was the youngest of three children, a factor which was, at a later date, thought to have considerable bearing on her speech behaviour.

Speech assessment

Data collected by picture naming was analysed using PACS (Grunwell, 1985b). It was found to be almost impossible to analyse

Syllable-initial, word-initial

Syllable-initial, within word

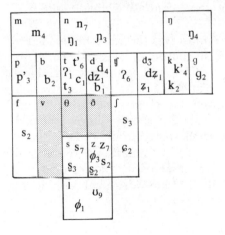

Syllable-final, word-final

Figure 7.1 The table shows the system of consonants in three word positions for single-word utterances. The subscripts refer to the number of occasions on which variant pronunciations were heard; thus, for target /m/ in SIWI position, five words were presented, two being pronounced with [h] and three with [ʔ]. Shaded areas indicate that no target was presented in assessment.

Table 7.1

Position in word	Number of target contrasts	Number of M's contrasts	*Number of phonetic variants
Syllable-initial, word-initial	19	0	7
Syllable-initial within word	19	9	30
Syllable-final, word-final	16	10	23

Note: *[Ø]: zero realization is counted as a single phonetic variant.

material collected in spontaneous connected utterances, since it was so often unglossable. There was felt to be no difference (significant to the planning of a remediation programme) between levels of intelligibility in single-word and connected-speech utterance. Figure 7.1 shows M's pronunciation of single-constant targets in three word positions. Table 7.1 summarizes the analysis revealing the gross reduction of system and marked phonetic variation in post-initial position. A striking feature of M's usage at this stage was the total lack of contrast in word-initial position, contrastive ability improving in subsequent word positions.

The disastrous lack of initial contrast was further compounded by a similar situation for word-initial consonant clusters, where the ubiquitous [?/h] realization was again found, with only occasional, but inconsistent, use of [b] for labial clusters. As for single sounds, realization of final clusters showed far greater maturity, though phonetic variation was present. Table 7.2 shows cluster pronunciations. (Only one occurrence of each cluster realization was recorded, unless otherwise indicated by a subscript numeral.) A number of realizations can be accounted for in terms of normal regional variation: for example, the vocalization of /l/ in word-final position is a normal feature of London English.

Other assessments

In the search for an explanation for M's speech disorder a number of further investigations were carried out. Little was revealed which could clearly point to a failure of processing at any one level; receptive language capacity, hearing ability and auditory discrimination all proved to be well within normal limits. Oral structure was normal and developmental milestones had been reached at expected ages. The only findings which could be regarded as significant were:

Table 7.2

Word-initial		Word-final	
Target cluster	*M's realization*	*Target cluster*	*M's realization*
/sp/	[ɸ] [b]	/nd/	[nd]₂
/st/	[ʔ]₂ [h]	/nz/	[nz] [ndz]
/sk/	[ʔ] [h]	/ndʒ/	[ndʒ]
/sl/	[ʔ]	/ŋk/	[ŋkʰ] [ŋk']
/str/	[ʔ]	/mps/	[mps]
/br/	[b] [h] [ɸ]	/ps/	[ps]
/bl/	[b] [ʔ]	/ts/	[ʔs] [ʔɕ]₂ [t'] [ts]
/pr/	[ɸ] [ʔ]		
/pl/	[h]	/ks/	[ks]
/dr/	[h]	/kt/	[k']
/tr/	[ʔ] [h]₂	/st/	[sː]
/kr/	[ʔ] [h]₂	/lz/	[ʊɸ]
/kl/	[kʰ]		
/fl/	[h]		

1　she was small and frail;
2　despite good concentration, she had difficulty in sitting still for any length of time, and was a little clumsy in refined hand–eye co-ordination tasks;
3　there was some slight hesitation in carrying out tongue movements, especially tongue-tip elevation;
4　though able to imitate all sounds in isolation and in CV, VC and VCV nonsense sequences, similar slight hesitation was observed in the assessment of diadochokinetic skills; rates were, however, not felt to be particularly low.

The conclusion drawn was that there was no aetiological factor which could be regarded as solely responsible for the gross failure of speech, and certainly no marked organic or neurological deficit. The mild clumsiness was felt to be an indication that at least an element of dyspraxia was present (Edwards, 1984, reports finding clumsiness of gross and/or fine motor movements in ten children among thirteen studied). This finding accorded with indications in the data of sequential planning difficulties, the presence of phonetic variability and ejective production in post-initial word positions. M had previously had some therapy and this may have masked more apparent signs of dyspraxia. Therapy had been primarily phonological, aimed at enhancing use of /b/, /p/ and /d/ oppositions in word-initial position. There was, as can be seen from the summary of speech assessment, no appreciable carry-over into spontaneous speech. It is important to say here, that M, when reminded of the need to produce an initial plosive in words with these sounds was able to do so readily and when her own 'open' forms were echoed back she would frequently self-correct. Reminders needed, however, to be constant, and were useful only in the production of single-word utterances.

THE PROGRAMME OF REMEDIATION

The therapist is frequently faced with cases such as M's; communication is failing and urgently requires attention and yet there is doubt as to the true diagnosis. In such cases a threefold approach is recommended containing elements of *articulatory facilitation, phonological therapy* to expand system and structures, and reinforcement by constant reference to *auditory input*. In what follows the importance of auditory input for M will be demonstrated.

The primary aim was to establish a limited system of consonants in word-initial position, since their lack was felt to be the major contributor to speech unintelligibility, firstly [m n b d w l], followed by [g f s p t]. For the purposes of this discussion only this part of the programme will be presented here in any detail. It can be viewed retrospectively in three major stages, which evolved from observation of her progress (or *lack* of it!) and reaction to therapy.

Stage I

Since M was readily able to articulate and discriminate target sounds in different phonetic contexts, so that she was able to produce nonsense sequences, CV, VC and VCV, for all the above targets, a phonological approach was first tried. When minimal pairs/sets were presented, failure of pronunciation was immediate, unless a prompt was supplied. This could be auditory, for example, presented with *arm* vs *farm* the therapist prompted [f], or visual; M was asked to look at vocal-tract shape. (Even for 'non-visible' sounds this was helpful.) Carry-over, despite repeated practice, was negligible, so that even immediately after a successful response, without further prompting the initial consonant was omitted. Furthermore, though she might be prompted to get one of a pair/set right, if no prompt was given for subsequent targets, initial consonants were omitted, or she perseverated on the first target consonant.

Stage II

Since minimal-pair confrontation had not been effective beyond ready articulation with prompting, it seemed that it was insufficiently powerful to cue for M a change to phonological usage. This raised the question as to whether in reality articulation was as easy in words as it appeared to be. In stage II, therefore, real words were presented, but the primary aim was to remove focus from *opposition* and concentrate on articulation in different *word* environments. To this end, pictures of words, all beginning with the same phoneme were selected for practice in rotation, but without reference to minimal pairs/sets; for example, one session *ball, book, bed, boy*, etc., the next *man, milk, monkey, moon*, etc., and so forth. These were used thus:

1   *Presented by therapist*: 'This is a book.'
2   *Selected by M*: Stimulus – 'Which is the book?'
3   *Produced by M with auditory prompt*: Stimulus – 'What's this? It's [b] ...'
4   *Produced by M with visual prompt*: Stimulus – 'What's this? Look! It's ...' Therapist points to own face.
5   *Produced by M without prompt*: Stimulus – 'What's this?'

This proved, as before, immediately successful up to the point at which the prompt was removed. The fifth stage was therefore dropped and when later introduced success gradually increased. There remained, however, a marked discrepancy between easy success in prompted responses and unprompted responses, which continued to fail much of the time. There was no appreciable carryover into controlled dialogue or spontaneous speech. A further difficulty of overlearning was encountered, in that when the changeover from one word list to another was made, M tended again to perseverate production; in other words, if the *ball, book, bag*, etc., list had been used, when the *man, milk, monkey*, etc., list was introduced, M tended to produce [bæn, bɪlk, 'bʌŋkɪ], etc. The question then arose as to how an essentially articulatory approach (albeit in meaningful context), combined as in this stage with accompanying auditory input, could be extended to incorporate the need to *change* articulation so that it became phonologically functional. To this end word lists of minimal pairs with two (and later three) different initial consonants were drawn up and used simultaneously, target words alternating, so that, for example, 1 above became: 'This is a mat, and this is a bat.' The same procedure as above was then followed. Thus, the bias had shifted back to the phonological, though emphasis was still chiefly on 'the right sound for *this word*'. Success, however, remained proportionate to the amount of prompting supplied. Although some of the earlier articulation for words was beginning to consolidate, in that M more often produced the *first* target word spontaneously correctly, she still failed to make the necessary change for any subsequent words, perseveration or omission resulting.

REASSESSMENT

M had by now been attending for six months. The fact that clinical pressures only allowed for a single one-hour session per week doubtless contributed to her lack of progress. None the less, the results of reassessment were disappointing; word-initial consonant usage showed minimal change, this having been throughout the focus of attention. Within-word and word-final systems had shown no expansion, but phonetic variability had decreased; usage had stabilized and within-word ejective productions were no longer present. This was somewhat encouraging (though rather infuriating since they had not been the direct target of therapy!), but lack of change in that area addressed in therapy required a re-evaluation of therapeutic approach.

Stages I and II can be summarized as follows:

Stage I: Minimal-pair confrontation;
Stage II: (a) articulation practice with emphasis on the *word* as the unit to facilitate; (b) articulatory change from one word to another.

Both these stages had been accompanied by the incidental auditory stimulation which is a part of any productive programme. M had always co-operated and appeared interested in activities; motivation was not seen as problematic. It seemed, however, impossible to find, through these means, a way to impress on her the need not merely to 'please teacher', but to alter her speech patterns for her own sake. She had lost her earlier withdrawal, and despite the fact that this led to an increase in the number of occasions on which she was misunderstood, there was no corresponding increase in communicative frustration; indeed, her confidence had increased. She had, as it were, become a passive partaker in a weekly exercise in 'good speech behaviour'. At the time of reassessment this passivity, coupled with lack of any generalization, led to the instigation of stage III.

Stage III

Directed by the reported success of Hodson and Paden's approach to remediation (1983) for children such as M, in which 'auditory bombardment' plays a major part, it was decided not merely to increase emphasis on auditory input, but to concentrate on input alone. A four-month period followed in which M was never requested to produce any target either as an articulatory exercise or in minimal-pair confrontation. Thus *all* emphasis on production was removed. Similar word lists as for Stage II were used in rotation, a single sound per session initially, and later two and three sounds were targeted. The words were incorporated into a number of activities and games, but each session began and ended with the therapist reading a fifteen-word list, whilst M was required to be still and listen.

Previously, M's mother had been asked to partake in her therapy, but it was not clear how valuable the home contribution had been; despite guidance, she remained diffident and often reported M's lack of co-operation. In stage III it was possible to give a clear and explicit set of instructions; a minimum of one reading of the word list each day was requested, other listening tasks being set when possible. M started full-time primary education at this time and the assistance of her teacher was also sought.

It is not possible in this single case to say that this stage of treatment was most dynamic *because of its nature* in promoting progress; it could be that added home and school stimulation were contributory, or that the earlier stages had begun to take effect. Whatever the dynamics of the components in M's treatment (and these are further discussed below), after six weeks she began spontaneously and without prompting to produce a notable increase of correct forms, despite the fact that these were not being directly sought. She was often observed during listening work, to make silent rehearsals, and she was heard on a number of occasions to produce what might be described as 'word babble'. For example, if for target /m/ an activity or story involving *man, milk, milkman* was underway, M was heard saying *man, pan, man, ban, fan, man*, etc. She began too to self-correct quite soon after emphasis had changed to input; although most words remained 'initially open' she would attempt to include initial sounds for major constituents in any utterance. After four months reassessment showed a marked increase in initial-sound usage, particularly [m b w d], but the others above, although less stable and subject to greater variability, were also present, this constituting a definite advance. Whilst auditory work was not abandoned, production work was gradually reinstated in increasing amounts.

The remaining six months of M's therapy and her progress can be briefly summarized. Components of both stages I and II were gradually reintroduced, but at no stage was direct emphasis on auditory input abandoned. When therapy sessions became primarily productive, M's class teacher continued supportive auditory work. Progress from the time of second reassessment was rapid. M's phonology had not been totally undeveloped at the outset, but it would seem that she had a 'frozen system' which had halted acquisition. As soon as, in stage III, the 'thaw' set in, rapid change occurred. Three interesting features should be reported:

1 As the initial consonant system expanded, sounds which had earlier been articulated correctly in therapy in words became subject to normal developmental phonological processes. For example, where previously M had readily articulated [d] vs [g] in word-initial position, velar targets were now fronted to alveolars. Similarly, she passed through stages when many first attempts at targets words produced a tendency to harmonize place of articulation, and to stop fricatives. It was as if, after articulatory practice (note her 'word babble'), supported by auditory input, periods of phonological adjustment were needed, these occurring rapidly relative to the previously slow onset of change. This tended to confirm the suspicion that M's difficulty lay in the area of motor planning (dyspraxia), which had inhibited quite specifically the development of word-initial oppositions. Once this articulatory barrier had been removed, ready speech praxis enabled acquisition to proceed, progression passing through the stages of normal acquisition, towards a functional phonological system.

2 As new targets in therapy became increasingly complex, to paraphrase Stampe (1979), they increasingly 'tried the restrictions of her speech capacity', struggle behaviour was noted. This had not been witnessed previously and was never persistent. She passed quickly through the need to establish an articulatory pattern, which could then be fitted into the expanding phonology. This supplied further evidence that difficulty in establishing the motor patterns associated with sounds and sound sequences was at the root of her disorder. Sufficient practice in therapy had enabled her to establish a system for coping with new speech movement, and she could then proceed with dispatch through articulatory practice to functional use.

3 The time of maximum change, when each week new ground was broken, coincided with the birth of her sister. An appreciable change in her motivation also occurred; though, as has been said, she was a willing client, now her participation changed from passivity to an almost fierce concentration. It had earlier been observed that her family tended to 'baby' her and this could, in the light of the change at this point, have constituted a covert acceptance (even encourage-ment) of her speech patterns, despite overt protestations to the contrary. Here then is an additional factor, together with the fact that M had been a term in school, which cannot be separated in its effect upon her progress.

At the time of writing M is in her fourth term at school. Her speech is no longer unintelligible, though difficult to understand at times and the flow of speech is marked by dysfluency, a further confirmation that a diagnosis of articulatory dyspraxia is fitting. Some initial conso-nant clusters are still subject to reduction, she uses only two places of articulation for word-initial fricatives, and she still produces some 'initially open' syllables, especially when excited. Post-initial sub-systems remain much as they were at the time of first reassessment, and it is likely that M will continue to require speech therapy for some time.

DISCUSSION

In the introduction the synergistic nature of speech and language processing is discussed. It is the author's belief that therapy is inefficient if it fails to acknowledge the interaction of the perceptual, phonological and articulatory levels. The natural wish to find a single area which can be demonstrated as failing, and which can then be targeted in remediation, had led to the tendency to compartmentalize levels of processing and their equivalents in breakdown, thus isolating one from the other. Furthermore, practice has tended to be based on two fallacious assumptions. First, that if a child can articulate sounds singly, in nonsense sequences and in words, there is no bar to their full phonological use. If the child's phonology is inadequate, but she is found to be able to produce sounds up to the level of 'in words', emphasis in therapy is immediately placed on phonological contrast. Second, that if a child can perceive sounds as different in minimal pairs, perception is adequate for speech acquisition. The situation in clinical practice is still frequently found in which input levels are largely ignored and regarded as not requiring specific therapeutic intervention, if the child performs adequately on speech-discrimination tests.

The author is making no claim that what is reported here is the result of controlled research; rather that M's case highlighted a number of issues which are as yet unresolved and provides a valuable vehicle for discussion of the 'state of the art'. There were numerous variables which were 'hidden' initially, which would be hard to allow for in a controlled research programme. For example, it was only after the birth of her sister, that the possible role of parental attitude was truly appreciated, and the uncertainty of diagnosis would have rendered a controlled programme of one kind or the other unviable. (Furthermore, in the current economic climate it is increasingly difficult to attract funding for large-scale research; single case studies may prove of increasing value in future.)

What insights can be gained from reviewing this case and those like her? In M a number of features co-occurred which crystallized the author's thinking, both in terms of current theoretical stances, and in their application in practice. If the case for a threefold approach is taken as acceptable, then the following facets of M's history can be argued in its favour.

1 *No clear diagnosis was possible*: such, as said, is frequently the case. If synergy is a reality, it is by no means certain that any single area of failure can be said to exist in individuals with described phonological breakdown. Thus, though the suspicion existed that articulatory dyspraxia was present, and no obvious dysarthria or vocal-tract movement failure was found, M showed great difficulty in translating articulation into phonology. Though dyspraxia may have been responsible originally for upsetting the path of development, its effect of 'freezing' phonological acquisition was profound, and it is clearly impossible to remove the passage of time and get back to origins. By the inclusion of both phonetic/articulatory and phonological components M was eventually able to incorporate enhanced speech praxis into the reorganization of her phonology.

2 *A direct phonological approach was ineffective*: articulation was accessed as adequate, but the assumption that it was therefore phonologically viable proved false. As mentioned above, fallacious arguments may lead to progressions of thinking which omit intermediate stages in their arrival at what are therefore incomplete conclusions. To assume that she could 'use', simply because she could 'do', overlooked her need for practice and the deeper establishment of

articulatory patterns. Such phonetic practice as sʰ
indulged in was closely akin to the sound play witn
phonological acquisition, as is suggested by the term 'w
assuming a phonological stance, the phonetic-practice ᴅᴇ...
found in normal acquisition is sometimes discounted, simply because
the child in question is older and beyond the age at which such
behaviour is normally found. If there is any sense in basing therapeutic programmes on patterns of normal development (which surely
there must be) then articulation practice may play a major role, and
approaches which are purely phonological may by-pass this need.

3 *Input training was paramount*: M's programme took into account
both articulatory practice and phonological usage, but not until input
training was included was a real shift in her speech seen. Children do
not learn to associate articulatory differences in language by being
presented with minimal pairs. Though confrontation with communicative inadequacy may be sufficient for some to bridge the gap
between articulation and phonology, generalization may still fail.
Certainly in M's case it was insufficiently powerful to bring about
behavioural change. By enhancing input, whatever the mechanisms of
perception involved, it would seem that M was able at last to appreciate the requirement being made of her and to 'make them her own'. If
Borden and Harris's supposition, quoted above, is correct, then its
application is supported by M's progress. Though it is readily
acknowledged that perception aids production, the converse, that
production aids perception, whilst possibly not dismissed, is infrequently the direct focus of clinical applications. For M repeated and
focused articulation practice may have been the key to her ability to
perceive contrastive use, so that when input was enhanced, thus
increasing the likelihood of appreciating particular sounds in the
general speech environment, she was able to perceive her *own*
erroneous patterns and begin to match them, back through articulation ('word babble') to phonological usage.

(Another application of this principle, that perception depends on
production, can be seen in the training of students in phonetic skills.
Where students are unable to perceive differences between closely
related sounds, it is only through their *own* production that they
become aware of narrow auditory differences.)

4 *Teaching versus acquisition*: M's 'good speech behaviour' has
been alluded to before. Despite teaching of articulatory and
phonological skills, M remained in a state lacking true acquisitional

:hange until the picture was completed by the essential input training. Thereafter, her progress needed simply to be guided as she proceeded to acquire new usage. Although the therapist may wish to apply a 'teaching' framework, particularly to children already familiar with the school situation, it is, none the less, impossible to impose new speech patterns from outside. The therapist can only offer alternatives and enhance by emphasis those areas which are failing. Thus M was observed, despite advanced articulatory ability, to go through, at least to some extent, patterns of normal phonological acquisition reflected in the observation of phonological processes in stage III.

The lessons learnt from reviewing this case critically can be summarized in the argument that it was the emphasis on input training that fulfilled a critical need, but that all three components were necessary in affecting change. Whether an immediate attack at the input level would have been efficacious must remain a matter of speculation. The contention is that, since articulation was possible at the outset (and phonologically was to an extent mature post-initially), input training could have bridged the gap between 'good speech behaviour' (i.e., ready articulation of sounds in words when aided by prompting) and true phonological absorption of articulatory patterns.

Other variables, such as the role played by parental attitude and the amount of clinical time available, are, though doubtless significant, of less immediate relevance here. One further factor in support of the inclusion of input training exists: namely, that parents and teachers may be diffident, unable or unwilling to carry out tasks outside the clinic because they feel they lack clear understanding of therapy. They can, however, be readily encouraged to support input training, which can be simply explained. Whilst some parents are anxious in production work lest they 'do something wrong', they will seldom feel uncomfortable about, for example, reading a word list, or sharing an alphabet book with their child.

SUMMARY

It is hoped that, by presenting this case in the framework of an argument which sees as central the synergy of perception, phonology and articulation, some of the difficulties acknowledged by students approaching so-called 'phonological disorders' will have been brought into focus. As has been said, the understanding of perceptual capacities and the differences between inter- and intrapersonal perception, are as yet not fully understood. The processes involved in their further interaction with output levels, and in the breakdown of output, are by no means clear. In the light of current understanding, however, closer attention to input in therapy would seem essential, if a move towards greater enlightenment is to be made. It may in future be possible to pinpoint levels of disorder more accurately and to understand their interactions within the whole. In the meantime, the tendency to discard one vogue for another should be guarded against, lest the valuable insights of history, however lacking in clarity they may be, are lost.

REFERENCES

Berko, J. and Brown, R. (1960) 'Psycholinguistic research methods', in P. Mussen, (ed.) *Handbook of Research Methods in Child Development*, New York: Wiley, 517–57.

Bountress, N.G. and Laderberg, C. (1981) 'A comparison of two tests of in N.J. Lass (ed.) *Speech and Language: Advances in Basic Research and Practice*, vol. IV, New York: Academic Press.

Borden, G.J. and Harris, K.S. (1980) 'Speech perception', in *Speech Science Primer*, Baltimore/London: Williams & Wilkins, 161–213.

Bountress, N.G. (1984) 'A second look at tests of speech-sound discrimination', *Journal of Communication Disorders* 17: 349–59.

Bountress, N.G. and Laderberg, C. (1981) 'A comparison of two tests of speech-sound discrimination', *Journal of Communication Disorders* 14: 149–56.

Edwards, M. (1984) *Disorders of Articulation. Aspects of Dysarthria and Verbal Dyspraxia*, Vienna/New York: Springer.

Eimas, P.D., Siqueland, E.R., Jusczyk, P. and Vigorito, J. (1977) 'Speech perception in infants', *Science* 171: 303–6.

Fawcus, R. (1980) 'The treatment of phonological disorders', in F.M. Jones (ed.) *Language Disability in Children*, Lancaster: MTP Press.

Goldman, R., Fristoe, M. and Woodcock, R. (1970) *The Goldman–Fristoe–Woodcock Test of Auditory Discrimination*, Circle Pines, Minnesota: American Guidance Service.

Grunwell, P. (1982) *Clinical Phonology*, London: Croom Helm.

Grunwell, P. (1985a) 'Comments on the terms "phonetics" and "phonological" as applied in the investigation of speech disorders', *British Journal of Disorders of Communication* 20: 165–70.

Grunwell, P. (1985b) *Phonological Analysis of Child Speech* (PACS), Windsor: NFER-Nelson.

Harris, J. and Cottam, P. (1985) 'Phonetic features and phonological features in speech assessment', *British Journal of Disorders of Communication* 20: 61–74.

Hawkins, P. (1985) 'A tutorial comment on Harris and Cottam', *British Journal of Disorders of Communication* 20: 75–80.

Hewlett, P. (1985) 'Phonological versus phonetic disorders; some suggested modifications to the current use of the distinction', *British Journal of Disorders of Communication* 20: 155–64.

Hodson, B.W. and Paden, E.P. (1983) *Targeting Intelligible Speech*, San Diego: College Hill Press.

Ingram, D. (1976) *Phonological Disability in Children*, London: Arnold.

Jaffe, M.B. (1984) 'Neurological impairment of speech production: assessment and treatment', in J. Costello (ed.) *Speech Disorders in Children*, San Diego: College Hill Press, 157–86.

Liberman, A.M., Harris, K.S., Hoffman, H.S. and Griffith, B.C. (1957) 'The discrimination of speech sounds within and across phoneme boundaries', *Journal of Experimental Psychology* 54: 358–68.

Locke, J. (1980a) 'The inference of speech perception in the phonologically disordered child. Part I: A rationale, some criteria, the conventional tests', *Journal of Speech and Hearing Disorders* 45: 431–44.

Locke, J. (1980b) 'The inference of speech perception in the phonologically disordered child. Part II: Some clinically novel procedures, their use, some findings', *Journal of Speech and Hearing Disorders* 45: 445–68.

Locke, J.L. and Kutz, K.J. (1975) 'Memory for speech and speech for memory', *Journal of Speech and Hearing Research* 18: 176–91.

McReynolds, L.V., Kohn, J. and Williams, G.C. (1975) 'Articulatory-defective children's discrimination of their production errors', *Journal of Speech and Hearing Disorders* 40: 327–38.

Milroy, L. (1985) 'Phonological analysis and speech disorders: a comment', *British Journal of Disorders of Communication* 20: 171–9.

Pronovost, W. (1974) *The Boston University Speech Sound Discrimination Test*, Cedar Falls, IA: Go-Mo Products.

Stampe, D. (1979) *A Dissertation on Natural Phonology*, ed. I. Hankamer, New York: Garland.

Weiner, F. (1981) 'Treatment of phonological disability using the method of minimal meaningful contrast: two case studies', *Journal of Speech and Hearing Disorders* 46: 97–103.

Wepman, J. (1958) *Auditory Discrimination Test*, Chicago: Language Research Associates.

Williams, L. (1974) 'Speech perception and production as a function of exposure to second language', unpublished doctoral dissertation, Harvard University.

Index

action words 72–3, 146
active learning 46–7
active role see cognitive theory;
  prosodic theory
adequacy/inadequacy, functional
  124–6; communicative 121–3;
  see also FLOSS
adult input and theories 19–20,
  23–4, 25, 28–9, 31; identification
  and reinforcement 19–20, 27, 31
africates: stopping see stops; see also
  liquids, fricatives and africates
aims see goals
Allen, G. 81
alliteration 100, 108
American English 142–51
amplification in treatment 146–7
analysis of disorders see
  characteristics; clinical-linguistics
anatomical factors see physiological
Anderson, J.M. 3
ankyloglossia 33
aphasia 18
APP see Assessment of Phonological
  Processes
apraxia, developmental see
  dyspraxia
articulation 20; and
  clinical-linguistics 39–40, 45, 51,
  52; and input training 153–4,
  157, 162–4, 166–7, 169
assessment 80, 143; and
  clinical-linguistic perspective
  49–59; goals 121–3, 133; and
  input training 154, 155, 156,
  158–62, 164–7; and
  metalinguistic awareness 113–14;

output and input in 155–7; see
  also clinical-linguistics; FLOSS;
  functional considerations
Assessment of Phonological
  Processes (APP) 50–2, 54, 56–7,
  143
assimilation 21–2, 45, 50, 52, 53,
  71, 145
asymmetricality 44
ATTEMPTED 71
auditory-perceptual component 32;
  discrimination see perception and
  rhyming; in input training 162,
  165, 166; problems see hearing;
  in treatment 145, 146, 147, 148
automaticity 76
awareness, linguistic 146; defined
  91–2, 108; see also metalinguistic
  awareness

babbling 71; and input training 155,
  158, 165, 169; and theories 18,
  19, 25–6, 27
backing 56, 144
Bankson, N. 10, 58
behaviourist theory 19–21, 27, 31
Benjamin, B.J. 57
Bennett, S. 10
Berko, J. 156
Bernhardt, B. 10
Bernthal, J.E. 58
Bertelson, P. 89
between-word errors 77–9
Bilger, R.C. 26
biological theory 16, 17, 25–6, 27,
  30, 31–2
Blache, S. 10